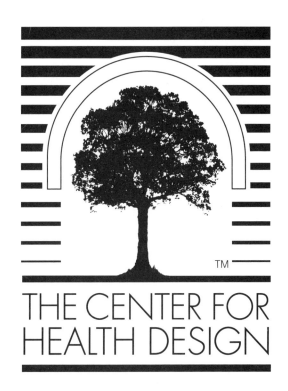

THE CENTER FOR HEALTH DESIGN

A GUIDE TO CONDUCTING HEALTHCARE FACILITY VISITS

by Craig Zimring, Ph.D.
Georgia Institute of Technology

Published by: The Center for Health Design, Inc.
Publisher: Wayne Ruga, AIA, ISID
Research Consultant: Craig Zimring, Ph.D., College of Architecture, Georgia Institute of Technology
Printer: Eusey Press

The Center for Health Design, Inc.
4550 Alhambra Way
Martinez, CA 94553
United States of America
Tel: (510) 370-0345
Fax: (510) 228-4018

Craig Zimring, Ph.D.
College of Architecture
Georgia Institute of Technology
Atlanta, GA 30332-0155
Tel: (404) 894-3915
Fax: (404) 894-1629
email: craig.zimring@arch.gatech.edu

First Printing, October 1994
ISBN 0-9638938-1-5
Printed in the United States of America

ACKNOWLEDGMENTS

The Center for Health Design would like to acknowledge the following individuals and organizations for making this research project possible.

Board of Directors
Russell C. Coile, Jr.
Ann Dix
David Guynes
Kathryn Johnson
Kerwin Kettler, IDEC
Roger K. Leib, AIA
Cynthia A. Leibrock, ASID
Debra J. Levin
Jain Malkin
Sara O. Marberry
Robin Orr, MPH
Derek Parker, FAIA, RIBA
James Ray, FACHE
Wayne Ruga, AIA, ISID

Research Committee
Janet R. Carpman, PhD
Uriel Cohen, D.Arch
Syed V. Husain
Debra J. Levin
M.P. MacDougall
Jain Malkin
James Ray, FACHE
David Reid
Wayne Ruga, AIA, ISID
Mardelle Shepley, D.Arch
Karen Tetlow
Roger Ulrich, PhD

Project Advisory Board
Ren Davis
Dennis Dunne
Dale Durfee, AIA
Larry Lord, FAIA
Leslie Saunders, AIA

Sponsors
This Research Report has been exclusively sponsored by: Armstrong World Industries, Milcare, Inc., and Thomasville Furniture.

Research Consultants
Georgia Institute of Technology
Craig Zimring, Ph.D.
Osman Ataman
Rhonda Hillman
Samia Rab

Anshen + Allen
Bruce Nepp, AIA
Lynn Befu

Graphics and layout by
Margaret Gilchrist Serrato
Lord, Aeck & Sargent

The research consultants would like to thank Wayne Ruga and Debra Levin for their constant support and thoughtful attention to this project.

We would like to acknowledge the following individuals for generously providing their time:

DESIGN PROFESSIONALS INTERVIEWED

Richard Babcock
Interior Designer, Henningson, Durham and Richardson, Inc., Omaha, NE

Greg Barker
Vice President, Jay Farbstein and Associates, San Luis Obispo, CA

Jim Brinkley
Principal, NBBJ, Seattle, WA

Lisa Bryant
Project Manager, Thompson Design Associates, Reno, NV

Tom Cardinal
Associate Programmer, CRSS, Atlanta, GA

Jon Crane
Architect, Lord, Aeck & Sargent , Atlanta, GA

Rusty Foster
Principal, Coleman and Foster Architects, Memphis, TN

Ralph Hawkins
Architect, HKS, Inc. Dallas, TX

Rick Hintz
Vice President, Hammel, Green and Abrahamson (HGA), Minneapolis, MN

Barbara Huelat
Principal Interior Designer, Huelat Parimucha Healthcare Design, Arlington, VA

Dennis C. LaGatta
Vice President, Ellerbe Becket, Washington, D.C.

Larry Lord
Principal, Lord, Aeck & Sargent, Atlanta, Georgia

Joanne MacIsaac
Vice President, Interior Design, TRO - The Ritchie Organization, Newton, MA

Larry M. Oppenheimer
Principal, O'Donnell, Wicklund, Pigozzi & Peterson, Inc., Deerfield, IL

Kenneth Ritchin
Kenneth Ritchin Architecture and Planning, Jericho, NY

William Sarama
Senior Healthcare Architect, SOM, New York, NY

Les Saunders
Architect, Nix, Mann and Associates, Inc., Atlanta, GA

Tommy Thompson
Medical Planner Architect, Sherlock, Smith and Adams, Montgomery, AL

Bennett Wiggins
Architect, Lord, Aeck & Sargent, Atlanta, GA

HEALTHCARE PROFESSIONALS AND ADMINISTRATORS INTERVIEWED

Sue Balderson
Emergency Department Coordinator, St. Joseph's Hospital, Parkersburg, WV

Georgia Brogdon
Vice President, Operations, Gwinnett Women's Pavilion, Lawrenceville, GA

James W. Evans
Facilities Director, Heartland Health System, St. Joseph, MO

Charles G. Farmer
Assistant Administrator Plant Operations, Arlington Memorial Hospital, Arlington, TX

Dewane K. Funderburg
Director, Physical Facilities, Arkansas Children's Hospital, Little Rock, AR

John L. Hoffman
Director, Facilities Planning, Carle Foundation Hospital, Urbana, IL

Kathy Hooper
Administrator, Ambulatory Care, Atlantic City Medical Center, Atlantic City, NJ

Mikhail Khlyavich
Director, Design and Construction, Mount Sinai Medical Center, New York, NY

Lewis Saylor
Vice President, Marketing, Bristol Regional Medical Center, Bristol, TN

Robert Terry
Director of Facilities Management, Emory University Hospital, Atlanta, GA

Jim Venker
Director, Facilities Development, Ochsner Foundation Hospital, New Orleans, LA

Marvina Williams
Director, Emergency Center , Kennestone Hospital, Marietta, GA

Bing G. Zillmer
Director of Engineering Service, Lutheran Hospital, La Crosse, WI

CONTENTS

INTRODUCTION

A major medical center is building a new diagnostic and treatment center that will include both inpatient services and expensive high technology outpatient services. The center is considering whether to provide day surgery within the diagnostic and treatment center or in a freestanding outpatient facility. They are facing a dilemma. If they locate the day surgery center separately, they can use lower-cost construction. If they combine the functions, they can use the spare capacity that will likely become available in the inpatient operating rooms. This is especially important as outpatient procedures become increasingly complex. The center wishes to evaluate sites that currently operate in fully separate facilities versus ones that provide separate outpatient and inpatient reception and recovery facilities, but share operating rooms.

A large interiors firm has been contacted to conduct a visit of several new children's hospitals in the Northwest. Eager to get the commission from this major hospital corporation to renovate the interior of a large children's hospital, the firm arranges visits of hospitals it has designed as well as two designed by other firms.

An architecture firm is renovating a large medical laboratory in an existing building which has a minimal 11-foot-3-inch floor-to-floor height. Concerned that the client may not understand the implications of this tight dimension—which means that the fume hood ventilation system can not easily be installed within this space—the architects arrange visits of other labs with similar floor-to-floor heights.

Change in healthcare and society is rapid and increasingly unpredictable, bringing an unprecedented level of risk for healthcare organizations facing new projects. This guide discusses a specific tool that healthcare organizations and design professionals can use to help manage uncertainty: the facility visit. In almost every healthcare project someone—client, designer, or client-design team—visits other facilities to help them prepare for the project. A probing, well structured, and well run visit can highlight the range of possible design and operational alternatives, pinpoint potential problems, and build a design team that works together effectively over the course of a design project. It can help a team creatively break their existing paradigms for their current project and can provide a pool of experience that can inform other projects. All of these can help reduce risk for healthcare organizations.

However, current facility visits are often ineffective. They are frequently conducted quite casually, despite the rigor of much other healthcare planning and design. Visits are often costly—$40,000 or more—yet they often fall short of their potential. Sites are often chosen without careful consideration, little attention is given to clarifying the purpose or methods of visits, there is often little wrap-up, and frequently no final report is prepared. Not only is the money devoted to the visit frequently not used most effectively, the visit presents important opportunities to learn and to build a design team. These opportunities are too often squandered.

This guide focuses on what a facility field visit can accomplish and suggests ways to achieve these goals. Although a facility visit may occur in a variety of circumstances, including the redesign of the process of healthcare without any redesign of the physical setting, this guide focuses on situations in which architectural or interior design is being contemplated or is in process.

SCOPE OF THE RESEARCH

The goals of this project were to learn about the existing practice of conducting healthcare facility visits, to learn about the potential for extending their rigor and effectiveness, and to develop and test a new approach. We interviewed over 40 professionals in the fields of healthcare and design from every region of the US, including interior designers, architects, and clients who had participated in design projects, and healthcare professionals who conduct visits of their own facilities. We sampled professionals from large and small design firms, and from large and small medical organizations. To get a picture of both "average" and "excellent" practice we randomly selected members from professional organizations such as the AIA Academy on Architecture for Health and the American Society of Hospital Engineers, and augmented these with firms and individuals who were award winners or were recommended to us by top practitioners. We developed a multi-page questionnaire that probed the participants' experiences with visits, including their reasons for participating, their methods, and how they used the information produced. We faxed each participant the questionnaire, then followed up with an interview on the phone or in person. The interviews averaged about one-and-a-half hours in length. Every person we initially contacted participated in an interview. Everyone in our sample had participated in some sort of visit of healthcare facilities within the past year.

After conducting the interviews we developed, field tested, and revised a new facility visit method, which is presented in this guide. Throughout this process we conferred with select members of the Research Committee of The Center for Health Design and the Project Advisory Board. (The members of these groups are listed in the Acknowledgments, above.)

GOALS OF FACILITY VISITS

There are many reasons for doing a facility visit and many different kinds of visits. However, visits roughly fall into three categories: specific visits, departmental visits and general visits. Specific visits focus on particular issues such as the design of patient room headwalls, nursing stations, or gift shops; departmental visits focus on learning about the operations and design of whole departments such as outpatient imaging or neonatal intensive care; general visits are concerned with issues relevant to a whole institution, such as how to restructure operations to become patient-focused. Usually, departmental and general visits occur during programming or schematic design; specific visits often occur during design development, when decisions are being made about materials, finishes and equipment.

More broadly, there are several general reasons for conducting visits: learning about state-of-the art facilities; thinking about projects in new ways; and creating an effective design team.

LEARNING ABOUT STATE-OF-THE-ART FACILITIES

Visit participants want to learn what excellent organizations in their field, both competitors and other organizations, are doing. Participants are often particularly interested in learning how changes in business, technology or demographics, such as increased focus on outpatient facilities or increased criticality of inpatients, might affect their own operations and design. For example, in Story 1, below, a UK team was interested in grafting US experience onto a UK healthcare culture. In another example, hospital personnel at Georgia's St. Joseph's Hospital visited five emergency rooms over the course of several weeks before implementing an "express" service of their own. According to planner Greg Barker (Jay Farbstein & Associates, CA) they "use site visits as a method of exposing the clients to a broader range of operating philosophies and methods." This gives the clients and design professionals a common frame of reference on which to base critical operational and design decisions.

STORY 1 William Headley, North Durham Acute Hospitals, UK

Traditionally, hospital design in the UK has been established centrally, with considerable emphasis placed on standard departmental areas and on a standardized planning format known as "Nucleus." The 20-year-old Nucleus system is based on a standard cruciform template of approximately 1,000 square meters housing a multitude of departments, which can be interlinked to provide the nucleus of a District General Hospital.

Durham wished to develop a hospital that in its vision would meet the challenges of the 21st Century, and produce a custom-designed hospital solution built to suit the needs of the patient, not just individual departments.

The brief has, therefore, to be developed from a blank sheet of paper and not from standard guidelines. It is also the Trust's objective to have the brief developed by staff from the bottom up. The purpose of the study tour was to allow frontline staff the opportunity to experience new ideas firsthand and talk to their medical counterparts about some of the philosophies of patient-focused care and to input their findings into the briefing process. We acknowledged the differences in the US and UK healthcare systems, but were interested in ensuring that best US practices, including the patient focused approach, facilities design, and the use of state of the art equipment, was studied and subsequently tailored to suit the new North Durham hospital.

THINKING ABOUT A PROJECT IN A NEW WAY

Participants who are currently engaged in a design or planning project are concerned with using visits to advance their own project. They use a visit to analyze innovative ideas and to help open the design team to new ideas. At the same time they are interested in building consensus on a preferred option. In Story 2, below, a hospital serves as a frequent visit host because it shows how special bay designs can be used in neonatal intensive care, and participants can consider how these designs apply to their current project. Other visit organizers see a visit as an opportunity for focusing the team on key decisions that need to be made, or to help the team focus in a systematic way on a range of strategic options and critical constraints. The visit exposes each team member to a variety of ways of accomplishing a similar program of requirements and thus starts the debate on how to achieve the best results for the facility being designed.

STORY 2 Georgia Brogdon, Vice President Operations, Gwinnett Women's Pavilion, GA

We get visitors at our facility about once per month. Right now the NICU (neonatal intensive care unit) is the most frequently visited location. The main reason is that Ohmeda uses our unit as a showcase for a special design of NICU bays. People want to see it because most think that Hill Rom is the only vendor of this type of equipment.

Early on, we were also one of the only state-of-the-art LDR facilities around. So if people wanted to visit an LDR unit, they had little choice but to come here. Now, however, people come to see us because we are a freestanding yet still attached facility. Over time the visits have evolved away from the design of the facility and more into programming, services, and operational issues.

We give three types of visits: 1) overview visits for lay people who just want to come see the area; 2) functional visits for other hospital people or architects who want to see the LDR design, mother/baby floor, NICU design, etc.; 3) operational flow visits to learn how the LDR concept impacts operations. In general, we start the visitors wherever the patient would start in the facility.

To arrange a successful visit of our facility, we need to know the interests of the visitors; then we can focus the schedule on that. Also knowing who they are bringing is helpful. You need to have their counterparts available. The types of information needed to conduct facility visits are: 1) what specific operational information to ask for in advance—size, number of rooms, number of physicians, staffing, C-section rate, whether they are a trauma center; 2) how to prepare for the visit; 3) who to bring. We've found that periodically the visitors are disappointed because they didn't bring enough people. Better to have too many than not enough.

CREATING AN EFFECTIVE DESIGN TEAM

Participants use visits as an opportunity for team building. Many visits are conducted early in a design project by a team who will work together for several years. The visit provides participants a useful opportunity to get to know each other and to build an effective team. As Story 3 illustrates, clients often look to a visit to see how well designers can understand their needs; designers use it as a way to learn about their clients and to mutually explore new ideas. A visit can also provide an opportunity for medical programmers to work with designers and clients. This is particularly important if programming and design are done by different firms.

Many visit participants focus on interpersonal issues: spending several days with someone helps build a personal relationship that one can rely on during a multi-year project. A visit also provides the opportunity to achieve other aspects of team building: clarifying values, goals, roles and expertise of individual participants; and identifying conflicts early so they can be resolved. One result for some teams is that it establishes a common vocabulary of operational and facility terms translated to the local healthcare facility.

STORY 3 Bing Zillmer, Director Engineering Services, Lutheran Hospital, La Crosse, WI

Conducting a facility field visit is an opportunity to have that one-on-one contact and find out if the architect "walks the talk or talks the walk." The biggest benefit is in finding out how the visit team of the architectural firm has been assembled: to see their level of participation, and how they have interacted with and listened to the clients and the hosts. What we look for in a consultant is not a "yes man"; we look for someone who knows more about existing facilities than we do. Our key concerns are how the team worked together, how they listened.

Dennis C. Lagatta, Vice President, Ellerbe Becket, Washington, DC

The main reason for conducting a visit is to settle an issue with the client. The clients usually have only two frames of reference: the current facility and the one where they were trained. These two frames of reference are hard to overcome without a visit. We conduct visits to help settle an issue between various groups within the institution. The visit process tends to be a good political way to illustrate a problem or a solution to a problem. A good example is when you have a dispute between critical care physicians and surgeons. Both parties may be unwilling to compromise. Usually a visit will be a good way to defuse this conflict.

James W. Evans, Facilities Director, Heartland Health System, St. Louis, MO

Responding to the question, what kinds of team-building activities were conducted before the actual visit took place? The functional space program stage is where you start building a team. Functional space programming is a narrative of what you want to do. If the programming includes a laboratory or some other specialty area, you would also want to have the consultant (if you are using one) involved in this process. Between blocks and schematics is when you want to go on any visits. By working together and staying together through big and small projects, you develop a lot of rapport and credibility.

Les Saunders, Nix Mann And Associates, Architects, Atlanta, GA

In the case of marketing visits, we try and present our unique abilities to our clients and to get to know each other better. Our visits are generally tailored to what the client group is trying to accomplish. Our functional experts will go on the visit so they can get to know the client and try to enhance "bonding."

Facility visits allow healthcare organizations and design professionals to address several important trends in healthcare.

- As competition for patients increases, healthcare organizations are becoming more customer-oriented.

- A visit allows a team to understand the experience of stakeholders who they do not currently serve, and to examine the design and operations of facilities that are more customer-oriented.

- Social changes are resulting in some stakeholder groups gaining importance, such as outpatients involved in more complex procedures, higher acuity inpatients, older people, or non-English speakers.

- A visit may allow a team to learn about the experience and needs of some groups who may be unfamiliar to some healthcare organizations or design professionals.

- A greater emphasis on efficiency and Total Quality Management is placing more importance on benchmarking and data collection.

- A visit can provide quantitative and qualitative data that support future decision making.

- Tighter budgets, shorter design and construction schedules and more complex projects are requiring design teams to form more quickly and work more effectively.

- A visit can be an effective tool for building a design team early in a design project.

FALLING SHORT OF THEIR POTENTIAL

In a design project, the client healthcare organization generally pays for a visit, either directly or as a part of design fees. Do healthcare organizations usually get good value for their investment? Do visits generally achieve their ambitious goals of learning about competition and change, moving the design project along, and building teams? We found very different answers. Despite the usual rigor of healthcare planning and programming, many current visits are very casual. Whereas some planners of visits do careful searches of available facilities to fit specific criteria, most choose sites to visit in other ways— sites participants happen to already know because they have been written about in magazines, or sites where there is a contact that someone on the team knows. Though these ways of choosing sites may be appropriate, they raise a question as to whether most participants are visiting the best sites for their purposes.

In many cases visit teams simply do not spend much time structuring the visit. Most teams do not even meet in advance to decide the major foci of the visit. We did not find many groups who use checklists or sets of questions or criteria when they go into the field. Whereas some teams compile the participants' notes, and one team actually created a videotape in a large project, most teams do not create any kind of written or visual record of their visit. Many teams hold no meeting at the end to discuss the implications of the visit, although many participants felt that they emerged in subsequent programming or design meetings.

Despite the apparent casualness of these visits, designers and clients alike almost without exception felt they were a valuable resource.

Simply visiting a well-run facility can be vivid and exciting. It is fascinating to see how excellent competitors operate, to talk to them and learn of their experience. (It is also an excellent opportunity for administrators and designers to get away from their daily routine and talk to professional counterparts.)

But there are large opportunity costs in the way most current visits are run, and they represent considerable lost value for the healthcare organization, designer, and design project.

COMMON PITFALLS

Opportunity costs of current visits come from several common pitfalls.

1. LOW EXPECTATIONS LEAD TO LIMITED BENEFITS
    Often, participants see field visits as a way to get to know other team members and simply to see other sites, but have no clear idea about what information can be helpful to the project at hand. They don't think through how the visit can help the goals of their project or organization.

2. TOO BUSY TO PLAN
    The planner of a visit faces multiple problems. Often the visit is seen as a minor part of the job of most participants and doesn't get much attention in advance; schedules and participants may change at the last minute. In many cases, no one is assigned to develop the overall plan of the visit, and to ask if the major components—choice of sites, choice of issues to investigate, methods for visits, ways of creating and disseminating a report—match the overall goals of the organization and project. This is especially ironic because participants are often advocates of careful planning in other areas.

3. TOO FOCUSED ON MARKETING
    Many visits, and especially designer-client visits, are billed as data gathering but are in fact aimed at marketing. A design firm may literally be marketing services or may be trying to get a client to accept a solution that they have already developed: marketing an idea. This may lead to an attempt to create a perfect situation in the facility being visited, one without rush, bustle, or everyday users and the information they can provide. For designer-client teams, we heard many designers complain that they couldn't control their clients, that they couldn't keep

them focused on prearranged ideas or keep them limited to prearranged routes. (This is often the result of not enough advance work aimed at understanding what interests the participants have and not enough time spent building common goals.)

4. CLOSING THE RANGE OF DESIGN OPTIONS TOO EARLY
    Many visits occur early in the design process or when an organization is considering significant change, a perfect time to consider new possibilities or address issues and solutions not previously considered. This timing, and the chance to see and discuss new options in a visit, presents an opportunity for a design team to open its range of choices and consider novel or creative alternatives. However, many visit participants feel strong pressures to "already know the answer" when they start the visit. Many designers and consultants feel that their clients do not want them to genuinely explore a range of options, that they were hired because they know the solution. Similarly, some medical professionals establish positions early to avoid seeming foolish or uninformed. As a result, the team may choose sites that bring only confirmation, not surprise, and people will be interviewed who bring a viewpoint that is already well established. This is not simply a matter of the individual personalities of people who set up visits, but rather a problem of the design of teams and the context within which they operate. It is often important for a design firm to show a client the approach it is advocating and for them to jointly explore its suitability for the client's project. However, if the client expects a designer to know the answer before the process starts, rather than developing it jointly with the client, the designer is forced to use the visit to exhort rather than to investigate.

5. TOO LITTLE STRUCTURE FOR THE VISIT
    Whereas no one likes to be burdened with unnecessary paperwork before or during a visit, it is easy to miss key issues if there is not an effort to establish issues in advance, with a reminder during the visit. Seeing a new place, with lots of activity and complexity, makes it easy to miss some key features. Many team members come back from visits with a clear idea of some irrelevant unique feature such as the sculpture in the hallway, rather than the aspect of the site that was being investigated.

6. INTERVIEWING THE WRONG PEOPLE

Often, out of organizational procedure or courtesy, a site being visited will assign an administrator or person from public relations to be the primary guide. It is almost always preferable to interview people familiar with the daily operations of the department or site.

7. MISSING CRITICAL STAKEHOLDERS

Almost every healthcare facility is attempting to become more responsive to customers, both patients and "internal" customers such as staff. Patients often now have a choice of healthcare providers, and staff are costly to replace. Despite these trends, many visits miss some key customer groups such as inpatients, outpatients, visitors, line staff, and maintenance staff. It is very important that these groups or people who have close contact with them be represented in visits.

8. A DESIGNER PROVIDING TOO MUCH DIRECTION DURING A DESIGNER-CLIENT VISIT

In an effort to control the outcome, a designer may attempt to ask most of the questions during interviews. In addition to the problem of focusing exclusively on "selling" ideas described above, clients do not like to feel that their role is usurped.

9. MISSING OPPORTUNITIES FOR TEAM BUILDING

Teams are most effective when everyone understands the values, goals, expertise and specific roles of others on the team. Teams are also most effective when the team understands the process and resources of the team, the nature of the final product, how the final product will be used, who will evaluate it, and by what criteria the success of the product will be evaluated. Although management consultants routinely recommend making such issues explicit at the beginning of team building, we found few visit teams that deal with these issues directly. Many teams do not even get together before a visit to discuss these issues.

10. NOT ATTENDING TO CREATING A COMMON LANGUAGE

Multidisciplinary design teams often speak different professional languages and have different interests and values. Designers are used to reading plans and thinking in terms of space and materials; healthcare administrators are used to thinking in terms of words and operational plans. Unless a field visit team is conscious about making links between space and operations, there can be little opportunity to establish agreement.

11. LACK OF AN ACCESSIBLE VISIT REPORT
Most current visits produce no report at all; some produce at least a compilation of handwritten notes. We heard a repeated problem: no one could remember where they saw a given feature.

Major Tasks

The healthcare facility visit process has three major phases, divided into specific team tasks that are conducted before, during, and after a visit. These phases, and the 13 major tasks that comprise them, are shown in Figure 1. The process we propose is quite straightforward, but compared to most current visits it is more deliberate about defining goals, thinking through what will be observed, preparing a report, and being clear about the implications of the visit for the current design project.

PREPARATION

1	Summarize the Design Project
2	Prepare Background Brief
3	Prepare Draft Work Plan and Budget
4	Choose and Invite Participants
5	Conduct Issues Session
6	Identify Sites — Start Site Visit Package
7	Confirm Agenda and Issues List
8	Complete Site Visit Package

SITE VISIT

9	Conduct Site Visit

FOCUS

10	Assemble Report Draft
11	Conduct Focus Meeting
12	Prepare and Distribute Focus Report
13	Use Data to Inform Design

Figure 1. Healthcare Facility Visit Process

PREPARATION

■ TASK 1. SUMMARIZE THE DESIGN PROJECT

In this task the project leader or others prepare a brief description of the goals, philosophy, scope, and major constraints overview of the design project that the visit is intended to aid. It should include the shortcomings that the design project is to resolve: space limitations, operational inefficiencies, deferred maintenance, etc.

The overview helps focus the facility visit, and can be provided to the host sites to help them understand the perspective of the visit. This summary should be brief, only a few pages of bulleted items, but should clearly identify the strategic decisions the team is facing. For example, a team may be considering whether to develop a freestanding or attached woman's pavilion. It is also important to identify key operational questions in the project summary. Focusing on design solutions too early may distract the team from more fundamental questions that need to be resolved. The purpose of the summary is to establish a common understanding of goals, build a common understanding of constraints, and allow the visit hosts to prepare for the visit.

The summary of the design project may focus on several topics:

- What deficiencies is the project trying to resolve?

- What is new or controversial about the project?

- Who are the key stakeholders? What needs or perspectives do they have, or what questions does the team have about these perspectives? A specific stakeholder list including "outpatients, family, maintenance staff" is often very useful; some key groups often get short shrift due to time or the experience of the team. This is particularly important if the team is changing healthcare philosophies and new groups such as outpatients are becoming more important.

- What are the critical purposes of the department or function being designed or renovated? For instance, a critical purpose of an operating room is to prevent infection during surgery; if the operating room does not achieve this purpose, it cannot serve as an operating room. By contrast, the waiting room outside does not have to prevent infection to achieve its purpose.

- What design or operational features relate to these critical purposes?

- How do these critical purposes link to key business imperatives, such as "broadening the base of patients" or "allowing nurses to spend more time delivering patient care"?

- What measurable or observable aspects of the design relate to these key purposes? For example, one team may be interested in whether carpeting leads to increased cleaning costs or increased infection rates; another team may be interested in visitor satisfaction with a self-service gift shop.

Key issues in summarizing the design project:

- It should be a brief synopsis that identifies key questions for the visit team and the host site.

- It should generally highlight operational questions.

- It should identify the full range of stakeholders who affect the current design.

Note: Many visits ignore this critical up-front work. Depending on the schedule and scope, the summary can be circulated to the team in advance of the brainstorming meeting.

■ TASK 2. PREPARE BACKGROUND BRIEF

More than most building types, healthcare facilities have a large body of literature providing descriptions of new trends, research, design guidelines, and post-occupancy evaluations. Many design firms and healthcare organizations have this material in their library or can get it from local universities or medical schools. In this task the visit organizer creates a file of a few key articles or book chapters describing the issue or facility type being visited. These are then distributed to the team, allowing all team members to have at least a minimal current understanding of operations and design.

The team leader also prepares an Issues Worksheet. This is a one-page form that is distributed along with the Background Brief to all members of the visit team prior to their first meeting. (See Figure 2 for a sample Issues Worksheet.) It encourages them to jot down what is important to them, and to discuss issues with their coworkers. It works most effectively when the visit organizer adds some typical issues to help them think through the problem. Participants should be encouraged to bring the Worksheet with them to the team meetings.

Key issues in preparing the Background Brief:

- Providing a few current background articles on the kind of department, facility, or process being visited helps create at least a minimum level of competence for the team and helps establish a common vocabulary prior to the visit.

- The Issues Worksheet, along with the Project Summary and Background Brief, allows participants to develop a picture of the project and to brainstorm ideas.

■ TASK 3. PREPARE DRAFT WORK PLAN AND BUDGET

Once the team leader or others have summarized the design project and prepared the Background Brief, a draft work plan outlining the major components of the field visits can be prepared. At this stage, it is important to establish a tentative budget for the visit. It is also important to make sure that the major components of the draft work plan, such as choosing visit sites and developing critical issues, match the overall goals of the organization and project. The draft work plan provides a tentative structure for the field visits, which can be modified by other team members.

Key issues in preparing the draft work plan:

- The work plan should restate how the visit will advance the design project.

- Budgets vary widely, but preliminary tasks and report writing often comprise one-third to one-half of the person-hours devoted to a visit. For example, it is not unusual for a three-day visit with seven people to require an additional 10 person-days or more to schedule the visit, coordinate with the sites, conduct the issues sessions, and prepare a simple draft report.

- In client-designer visits the client normally pays for the cost of its staff directly; a design firm will pay for its staff, but as reimbursable expenses these costs will be added onto the project costs.

ISSUES WORKSHEET

Department Level

Focus	LDRP		Name	Virginia Johnston, AIA
Date	7/15/94		Firm	King, Art & Major

TYPICAL ISSUES

Preprinted items prompt specific questions

- mission
- type of facility
- affiliation
- off-campus services
- main funding sources
- nature of patient
- list of departments
- # beds

QUESTIONS	RESOURCE	ISSUE TYPE	
	person or item	design	operational
What finish materials have been used successfully in the LDR room?	head nurse, facilities	☒	☐
How was the need for various lighting levels addressed in the the LDR rooms?	nurse, md facilities	☒	☐
Does the layout of LDR rooms in relation to the Nurses Station work effectively?	nurses	☒	☒
		☐	☐
		☐	☐
		☐	☐
		☐	☐
		☐	☐
		☐	☐
		☐	☐
		☐	☐
		☐	☐
		☐	☐

Area to record questions and issues

Place to identify resources

Type of issue

Figure 2. Issues Worksheet. Form used by participants to identify issues prior to the issues session.

■ TASK 4. CHOOSE AND INVITE PARTICIPANTS

The effectiveness of the team is, of course, most directly related to the nature of the participants. Field visit teams are sometimes chosen for reasons such as politics, or as a reward for good service, rather than for their relevance to the project. For healthcare organizations field visit teams are usually most successful if they mix the decision makers who will be empowered to make design decisions with people who have direct experience in working in the area or department being studied. For design firms, teams are often most successful if they include a principal and the project staff. In both of these cases, the team combines an overall strategic view of the organization and project with an intimate knowledge of operational and design details.

Key issues in choosing participants:

• Participants should be chosen with a clear view of why they need to participate and what their responsibility is in planning, conducting and writing up the visit.

• Site hosts say that teams larger than about seven tend to disrupt their operations.

■ TASK 5. CONDUCT TEAM ISSUES SESSION

It is usually advisable to hold a team meeting early in the visit planning process to: 1) clarify the purposes and general methods of the field visit; 2) build an effective visit team by clarifying the perspective and role of each participant; 3) identify potential sites, if the visit sites have not already been selected. Some resources and methods to select sites are discussed further in the next section, "Critical Issues in Conducting Facility Visits."

The issues session is often a "structured brainstorming" meeting aimed at getting a large number of ideas on the table. (This is particularly important during departmental and general visits, and if team members don't know each other.) The purpose is opening the range of possible issues rather than focusing on a single alternative.

This meeting is typically aimed at building a common sense of purpose for all team members, rather than marketing a preconceived idea. This meeting also serves the purpose of making critical decisions regarding the choice of sites and identifying who at the sites should be contacted.

Each participant should bring his or her Issues Worksheet along to the meeting. The initial task is to get all questions and information needs onto a flip chart pad or board before any prioritization goes on. Then the leader and group can sort these into categories and discuss priorities. These categories and priorities may be sorted in the form of lists which include: 1) a list of critical purposes of the departments or features being designed; 2) a list of critical purposes of the departments or features being evaluated at each facility during visits; 3) a list of existing and innovative design features relevant to these purposes. The critical purposes of the departments or design features at existing facilities can be charted at different spatial levels of the facilities, such as: site, entrance, public spaces, clinical spaces, administrative and support areas. Some typical architectural design issues are provided in the appendix.

The issues session may be run by the leader or the facilitator. Because one of the purposes of this meeting is to get balanced participation, it may be useful to have someone experienced in group process run the meeting, rather than the leader. His or her job is to make sure everyone participates, allowing the leader to focus on content.

This meeting may also provide an early opportunity to identify potential problems in conflicting goals, values or personalities on the team. For instance, a healthcare facility design project may have significant conflicts between departments, or between physicians and administrators. The meeting may also allow the team to agree on basic business imperatives and to be clear about the constraints that are of greatest importance to them, such as "never having radioactive materials cross the path of patients."

Key points in running an issues session:

• Everyone should be able to participate without feeling "dumb."

- The leader and group should try to understand the range of interests and priorities represented.

- Brief notes of the meeting should be distributed to all participants.

Note: This meeting is successful if participants feel they can express ideas, interests, and concerns without negative consequences from other members of the team. There is no such thing as a stupid question in this meeting.

■ TASK 6. IDENTIFY POTENTIAL SITES AND CONFIRM WITH THE TEAM

Based on the work plan which established the visit objectives and the desires, interests and budget of the team, the visit organizer chooses potential sites, and checks with the team. If possible, he or she provides some background information about each site to help the team make decisions.

The team may know of some sites they would like to visit, and these might have emerged in the issues session. Otherwise there are a range of sources for finding appropriate sites to visit: national organizations such as the American Hospital Association, as well as the American Institute of Architects Academy on Architecture for Health Facilities, and a range of magazines that discuss healthcare facilities. (See the section below entitled "Choosing Sites.")

Different teams pick sites for different reasons. Some may pick a site because it is the best example of an operational approach such as "patient-focused care." Others may look for diversity within a given set of constraints, such as different basic layouts of 250-bed inpatient facilities.

Many visit leaders complain that the team sometimes is distracted by features outside the focus of the tour, and particularly by poor maintenance. Wherever possible, it is advisable for the visit organizers to tour the site in advance of the group visit and to brief the hosts in person about the purposes of the visit. Although it is rare, some sites now charge for visits.

A key issue in choosing sites:

- The selection of sites should challenge the team to think in new ways.

Note: Sites are often chosen to provide a clear range of choices within a set of constraints provided by operations, budget, or existing conditions, such as "different layouts of express emergency departments" or "different designs of labor-delivery-post-partum-recovery rooms."

■ TASK 7. SCHEDULE SITES AND CONFIRM AGENDA

The leader or facilitator calls a representative at each host site to schedule the visit. He or she confirms the purposes of the visit, confirms with the host sites the information needed before and during the field visit, and confirms who will be interviewed at the site. Healthcare facilities are sometimes more responsive to a request for a visit if they are called by a healthcare professional or administrator rather than a designer: if someone on the team knows someone at a site, he or she may want to make the first phone call. Many teams also find that if they arrange for a very brief visit, this may be extended a bit on site when the hosts become engaged with the team. When confirming the schedule for the visit with the host facilities, the visit organizer should specify that the visit team would prefer to interview people familiar with the daily operations of the department or site.

Key issues in scheduling sites:

- Healthcare staff at the host facility prefer to know in advance who will participate on a visit, the purpose of the visit, and what information the team requires.

- Many sites feel that mid-morning or early afternoon visits are least disruptive to their housekeeping and medical rounds schedules.

Note: Sites are often proud of their facilities and often enjoy receiving distinguished visitors. However, they often find it difficult to arrange interviews or assemble detailed information on the spot.

■ TASK 8. PREPARE FIELD VISIT PACKAGE

Visits are more effective if participants are provided a package of information in advance: information about schedule, accommodations, and contact people; information about each site, including, where possible, brief background information and plans; a simple form for recording information; and a "tickler" list of questions and issues.

a) Prepare visit information package

The organizers should provide participants information about the logistics of the field visit: schedules, reservation confirmation numbers, phone numbers of sites and hotels.

b) Prepare site information package

The site information package orients participants to the site in advance of the visit. Depending on what information is available, it may include: plans and photos of each site; basic organizational information about the site (client name and address, mission statement, patient load, size, date, designers, etc.); description of special features or processes or other items of interest. Whereas measured plans are best, these are not often available. Fire evacuation plans can be used. A sample site information package is provided in the Appendix. Many teams find it useful to review job descriptions for the host site, and many organizations have these readily available.

c) Prepare Visit Worksheet

Facility visits are often overwhelming in the amount of information they present. It is useful for the organizers to provide the participants with a worksheet for taking notes. We have provided a sample worksheet as Figure 3 below, and blank forms are provided in the Appendix. The purpose of the checklist is to remind participants of the key issues and to provide a form that can easily be assembled into the trip report.

Note: A successful worksheet directs participants to the agreed-upon focal issues without burdening them with unnecessary paperwork. Participants should understand the relationship between filling out the checklist and filling out the final report.

HEALTHCARE FACILITY VISIT WORKSHEET

Name	Virginia Johnston, AIA	Date	July 29, 1994
Site	Metropolitan Hospital	Keywords	LDR, Labor Delivery Recovery, Maternity
Area	LDR		

ISSUES CHECKLIST

Programmatic / Operational
❏ what were the general operational issues to which the architecture of the facility directly responded?

❏ how does the facility function in terms of staff and administration?

❏ how is the facility staffed?

❏ security procedures

Special Features

❏ disinfecting Jacuzzi

❏ lighting in LDR

❏ how were special issues resolved?

Preprinted summary from Issues Worksheet

Plan and space for notes

OPERATIONAL/DESIGN ISSUES

Place to record other issues that arise during visit

Photo taken on visit

Figure 3. Healthcare Facility Visit Worksheet. Form used by participants during facility site visit.

FACILITY VISIT

■ TASK 9. CONDUCT FACILITY FIELD VISIT

The actual site visit typically includes: 1) an initial orientation interview with people at the site familiar with the department or setting being investigated; 2) a touring interview where the team, or part of it, visits the facility being investigated with someone familiar with daily operations, asking questions and observing operations; 3) recording the site; 4) conducting a wrap-up meeting at the site. (Each of these steps is discussed individually below.) The interview sessions are focused on helping the team understand a wider range of implications and possibilities. If appropriate, the wrap-up session may also be used for focusing on key issues that move the design along.

Note: Participants often like to speak to their counterparts: head nurse to head nurse, medical director to medical director, etc., although everyone seems to like to talk to people directly involved with running a facility such as a head nurse. People who know daily operations are often more useful than a high-level administrator or public relations staff member.

a) Conduct site orientation interview

During the orientation interview the visit team meets briefly with a representative of the site to get an overall orientation to the site: layout and general organization; mission and philosophy; brief history and strategic plans; patient load; treatment load; and other descriptions of the site. Many teams are also interested in learning about experiences the healthcare organization had with the process of planning, design, construction and facility management: What steps did they use? What innovations did they come up with? What problems did they encounter? What are they particularly proud of? What do they wish they had done differently?

b) Conduct a touring interview

The touring interview was developed by a building evaluation group in New Zealand and by several other post-occupancy evaluation researchers and practitioners. (See the post-occupancy evaluation section of the Bibliography.) In the touring interview, the team, or a portion of it, visits a portion of the site to understand the design and operations. Conducting an interview in the actual department being discussed often brings a vividness and specificity that may be lacking in an interview held in a meeting room or on the phone. One of the great strengths of the touring interview is the surprises it may bring, and the option it provides to consider new possibilities or to deal with unanticipated problems. As a result, it often works best to start with fairly open-ended questions:

- What works well here? What works less well?

- What are the major goals and operational philosophy of the department?

- What is the flow of patients, staff, visitors, meals, supplies, records, laundry, trash?

- Can they demonstrate a sample process or procedure, such as how a patient moves from the waiting room to gowning area to treatment area?

- What are they most proud of?

- What would they do differently if they could do it over?

These questions also provide a nonthreatening way to discuss shortcomings or issues that are potentially controversial. The team may then want to focus on the specific concerns that were raised in the issues session.

A difficult, but critically important, thing to avoid in a touring interview is to become distracted by idiosyncratic details of the site being visited. Often operational patterns or philosophy are more important than specific design features that will not be generalized to a new project: how equipment is allocated to labor-delivery-recovery-postpartum rooms in the site being visited may be more important than the color scheme, even though the color may be more striking.

Large multidisciplinary teams are particularly hard to manage during a touring interview. A given facility may have a state-of-the-art imaging department that is of great interest to the radiologists on the team but may have a mediocre rehabilitation department. In these cases, some of the touring interviews may be focused on "what the host would do differently next time."

Key issues in conducting the touring interview:

- Questions typically move from the general to the specific.

- The team should use what they see in the facility as an entrée into more focused questions.

- The recorders or all participants should keep notes to report back to the whole group.

Note: It is important to include people familiar with daily operations on the touring interview, both on the team side and on the side of the site being visited. A frequent problem is that some stakeholder groups such as patients or visitors are not represented; special efforts should be taken to understand the perspectives of these groups.

c) Document the visit

The goals of the visit dictate the kinds of documentation that are appropriate. However, most visits call for a visual record, sketches, and written notes.

In most cases it is useful to designate one or more "official" recorders who will assemble notes and be sure photos are taken, measurements made, plans and documents procured, etc. For designer-client visits, it is often useful to have at least two official recorders to look after both design and operational concerns. However, because a team often splits up, most or all participants may need to keep notes.

It is quite rare for teams to use video to record their visit, although this seems to be increasing in popularity. Editing videos can be very costly: it may take a staff member several person-days in a professional editing facility to edit several hours of raw video down to a 10- or 15- minute length. However, this time may be reduced with the increased availability of inexpensive microcomputer-based editing programs.

Key issues in recording the facility:

- Most visit participants find it useful to have clear plans of the facility or department they are visiting. Whereas some sites may not have these available, even fire evacuation plans can be used.

- Most participants find it useful to have labeled photographic prints of major spaces and features available as reminders later in the design process.

- Many departmental and general visit teams find it useful to photographically record key flows, such as patients, staff and supplies, and location of waiting rooms and other patient amenities.

Note: If the method of creating the documentation is established in advance it can easily be assembled into a draft report.

d) Conduct on-site wrap-up meeting

Whereas the visit interview is focused on opening options for the team and identifying new problems and issues, the wrap-up meeting is often more focused on clarifying how lessons learned on the visit relate to the design project, and how they begin to answer the questions the team established. It is often useful to have a representative of the host site present at the wrap-up meeting to answer questions, if their time allows.

Key issues in conducting wrap-up meetings:

- During the on-site wrap-up meeting the team may want to go around the room and solicit key observations and questions. In particular, if the team split up during the touring interview it is quite important to hear others' experiences.

- The recorders should keep track of key observations or questions, which become part of the visit report.

FOCUS

■ TASK 10. ASSEMBLE DRAFT VISIT REPORT

A draft visit report may take many different formats. The simplest is to photocopy and assemble all participants' worksheets and notes, retyping where necessary. Alternatively, the organizers or a portion of the team may edit and synthesize the worksheets and notes. Though more time consuming, this usually results in a more readable report. A somewhat more sophisticated version is to establish a database record that resembles the form used to take notes on-site in a program such as FoxPro, Dbase, or FileMaker Pro. Participants' comments can be typed into the database and sketches and graphics can be scanned in and attached. These are then provided to all participants.

A key issue in assembling the draft report:

• Simplicity is often best; simply photocopying or retyping notes is often adequate, especially if photos and sketches are attached.

■ TASK 11. CONDUCT FOCUS MEETING

Upon returning home, the team conducts a meeting to review the draft trip report and to ask:

• What are the major lessons of the visit?

• What does it tell the team about the current project?

Unlike the issues session held early in the visit planning process, which was primarily concerned with bringing out a wide range of goals and options, this meeting is typically more aimed at establishing consensus about directions for the project.

A key issue in conducting the focus meeting:

• The purpose of the focus meeting is to establish the lessons learned for the design project.

Note: The leader should carefully consider who is invited to the focus meeting. This may include others from the design firm, consultants, healthcare organization, or even representatives from the site.

■ TASK 12. PREPARE FOCUS REPORT

The focus report briefly summarizes the key conclusions of the visit for the visit team and for later use by the entire design team. It is an executive summary of the visit report which may provide a number of pages of observations and interview notes.

Key issues in preparing the focus report:

• The focus report should be a clear, brief, jargon-free summary.

■ TASK 13. USE DATA TO INFORM DESIGN

The key purpose of a facility visit is to inform design. Whereas this can occur informally in subsequent conversations and team meetings, it is best achieved by also being proactive. For example, the team can:

• Conduct an in-house feedback session about the visit.

• Create a database that is usable by the design team and others.

• Write a brief newsletter about the design project that includes key findings from the visit.

Key issues in using data to inform design:

• Reports and materials collected on visits should be available to all participants in the design process and should be on hand during subsequent meetings.

• A central archive of materials should be available and should be indexed to allow easy access for people involved in future projects.

TOOL KIT

TASK CHECKLIST

PREPARATION

■ TASK 1. SUMMARIZE THE DESIGN PROJECT

The team leader prepares a brief summary of the goals, philosophy, scope, and major constraints of the design project to help focus the field visit.

❑ Clarify what information is needed for the project.
❑ Summarize deficiencies the current design project is to resolve.
❑ Prepare a list of critical purposes of department or function being designed or renovated.
❑ Prepare a list of design or operational features related to these critical purposes.

■ TASK 2. PREPARE BACKGROUND BRIEF

The team leader prepares a file of a few key articles or book chapters that provide descriptions of new trends, research, design guidelines and post-occupancy evaluations of the facility type, department or issue being studied. He or she also prepares Issues Worksheets for team members to make notes on prior to the initial issues brainstorming session.

❑ Assemble current literature on existing facilities.
❑ Prepare the Issues Worksheet.

■ TASK 3. PREPARE DRAFT WORK PLAN AND BUDGET

The draft work plan clarifies the values, goals, process, schedule and resources of the visits.

❑ Outline major components of the facility visits with reference to the summarized design project and the Background Brief.
❑ Prepare a tentative budget for the field visits.

■ TASK 4. CHOOSE AND INVITE PARTICIPANTS

In this task the team leader builds a team. The ideal team combines a view of the overall strategic perspective of the organization and project with an intimate knowledge of daily operations.

❑ Prepare a list of visit participants.
❑ Send invitations to selected team members.
❑ Prepare a preliminary list of critical issues that need to be discussed in the team issues session.
❑ Prepare and distribute Issues Worksheets to team members.
❑ Distribute Background Brief to team members.

■ TASK 5. CONDUCT TEAM ISSUES SESSION

The team issues session has three purposes: 1) clarify the purposes and general methods for the field visit; 2) build an effective team; 3) identify potential sites. The issues session is often a "structured brainstorming" meeting aimed at getting a large number of ideas on the table, and at understanding the various perspectives of the team.

❑ Provide a summary of the design project to team members.

❑ Clarify the purpose, scope, and methods of the facility visit.

❑ Clarify the resources available to the team and the use of the information collected.

■ TASK 6. IDENTIFY POTENTIAL SITES AND START FACILITY VISIT PACKAGE

Based on visit objectives and the desires, interests and budget of the team, the visit organizers choose potential sites and check with the team. If possible they provide some background information about each site.

❑ Conduct a literature search for comparable facilities.

❑ Prepare preliminary fact sheets for potential sites.

❑ Confirm list of potential sites with participants.
    OR

❑ If field investigation sites are already selected, provide fact sheets about each site to the participants.

■ TASK 7. SCHEDULE SITES AND CONFIRM AGENDA

In this task, the purposes and schedule of the visit are confirmed with the sites. This should occur at least two weeks before the visit.

❑ Send overview of the design project and purpose of investigation to host sites.

❑ Determine information needed in advance and what is needed at arrival, and communicate this to host sites.

❑ Send issues and concerns of the visit to the host sites.

❑ Provide the host sites with names, phone numbers, description of roles and interests of all team members.

❑ Decide which representatives from the site facility are requested to participate in the investigation and the wrap-up meeting, and communicate this to the host sites.

❑ Ask about the policies for recording or photographing on the host sites.

■ TASK 8. PREPARE FIELD VISIT PACKAGE

The field investigation package includes the following components, which are used for conducting the visit:

❑ Tour information package (tour itineraries, transportation and accommodation details, list of contact people at each facility).

❑ Site information package (description of the sites, background information, facility plans).

❑ Site Visit Worksheets for notetaking.

SITE VISIT

■ TASK 9. CONDUCT FIELD VISIT

The interview sessions are focused on opening: helping the team understand a wider range of implications and possibilities. If appropriate, the wrap-up session may also be used for focusing on key issues that move the design along.

❑ Conduct site orientation interview.

❑ Collect any additional information from the host site.

❑ Conduct touring interview with people familiar with daily operations and a range of stakeholders.

❑ Document the visit through notes, sketches and photos.

❑ Conduct on-site wrap-up meeting with team members.

FOCUS

■ TASK 10. ASSEMBLE DRAFT VISIT REPORT

The draft report is a straightforward document allowing others to benefit from the investigation and providing the team a common document to work from.

❑ Send thank-you notes to contacts at site facilities.

❑ Consolidate field notes from Site Visit Worksheets.

❑ Extract key conclusions.

■ TASK 11. CONDUCT FOCUS MEETING

The team conducts a focus meeting to ask: What are the major lessons of the investigation? What does it tell the team about the current project?

❑ Confirm completeness of Draft Visit Report.

❑ Derive key conclusions of investigation.

❑ Develop action recommendations for design project.

■ TASK 12. PREPARE FOCUS REPORT

The Focus Report briefly summarizes the key conclusions of the visit for the visit team and for later use by the entire design team. It is an executive summary of the Visit Report which may provide a number of pages of observations and interview notes.

❏ Prepare and distribute a brief Focus Report.

■ TASK 13. USE DATA TO INFORM DESIGN

The purpose of this document is to inform the design process.

❏ Conduct in-house feedback sessions about the visit.

❏ Create a database that is usable by the design team and others.

❏ Write a brief newsletter about the design project that includes key findings from the visit.

SAMPLE FACILITY FACT SHEET

GWINNETT WOMEN'S PAVILION
SCHEDULED VISIT   Thursday, August 4, 1994
                              11:00 am

NAME: GWINNETT HOSPITAL SYSTEM
ADDRESS: Women's Pavilion
                           700 Medical Center Boulevard
                           Lawrenceville, GA 30245

CONTACT   Georgia Brogdon
                           Vice President, Operations
                           Gwinnett Women's Pavilion

TELEPHONE   (404) 822-6006   FAX (404) 822-6005

FACILITY DESIGN PROFESSIONALS
* Architect
  Nix Mann & Associates, 1382 Peachtree Street, NE, Atlanta, GA 30309

* Contractor
  R. J. Griffin & Company, 5775 Peachtree-Dunwoody Road, Suite 400C, Atlanta, GA 30342

* Interior Designer
  Hayden & Associates, 110 Industrial Park Drive, Lawrenceville, GA 30245

* Construction Consultants
  Causey & Associates, P. O. Box 7874, Macon, GA 31209

* Furnishing Suppliers
Office Desk	Creative Dimensions
Dad's Chair	Grand Manor
Lobby Seating	Vecta
Patient Bed	Hill Rom

* Equipment Suppliers
LDR Delivery Light	Berchtold Corp. (Martin USA)
LDR Bed	Hill Rom
Armoire	LIC Care
Bassinet	LIC Care
Infant Care Station	LIC Care
Bedside Monitor Table	LIC Care
Night Stand	LIC Care
NICU Headwalls	Ohmeda

SAMPLE FACILITY FACT SHEET

GWINNETT WOMEN'S PAVILION

BACKGROUND BRIEF

The Gwinnett Hospital System is a 391-bed facility located in Gwinnett County, north of Atlanta. The Hospital System includes:

1. Gwinnett Medical Center-190 beds, general acute care facility
2. Joan Glancy Memorial Hospital-90 beds, general acute care and inpatient rehabilitation
3. Gwinnett Treatment Center-24 beds, inpatient adult and adolescent substance abuse and psychiatry
4. Gwinnett Day Surgery-10 outpatient operating rooms
5. Gwinnett Women's Pavilion-34 beds

The Gwinnett Women's Pavilion is an LDR facility constructed in response to the volume increase and capacity problems in annual deliveries. It was designed as a freestanding facility connected to the main hospital by a bridge and a long corridor. The following services are located in the facility:

1. Nursing Station
    11 LDRs with Central Fetal Monitoring
    2 Obstetrical Operating Rooms
    8-Bed Recovery Room
    1 NST Lounge
    8-Exam/Triage Rooms
    2 Antepartum High Risk Rooms
    34 Private Postpartum Rooms
    40 Well Baby Beds
    2 Family Rooms
    16 Level III NICU beds

2. Diagnostic Services
    2 Dedicated Mammography Units
    2 Dedicated Ultrasound Units for Inpatients and Outpatients
    Lab Drawing Station for outpatients, women and infants only
    Amniocentesis
    Bone Density

3. Educational Services
    Comprehensive Perinatal Education
    Women's Night Out Lectures Series and Support Groups

SAMPLE FACILITY FACT SHEET

GWINNETT WOMEN'S PAVILION

4.   Respiratory Care Services
      Resuscitation Team Support
      Blood Gas Lab and NICU Ventilator Management
      Neonatal Transport Team

The Gwinnett Women's Pavilion operates 24 hours per day as a unit of the Gwinnett Medical Center.

Medical Staff Members
Obstetrics and Gynecology 12
Pediatricians 14
Anesthesiologists 8
Radiologists 8

SAMPLE FACILITY FACT SHEET

GWINNETT WOMEN'S PAVILION

GROUND FLOOR
The lobby and main entrance includes a waiting area, the reception desk, three admitting booths, a gift shop, and a playroom for children. Following services and activities are located on the ground floor:
- Education Offices (3), Classrooms (2), a Medical Records Storage Room.
- 10 LDR Rooms that are furnished in an attractive decor to create a warm, relaxed setting with a sitting area, Jacuzzi tub, an overstuffed chair for Dad that converts to a twin-size bed, and an armoire holding a television. The room easily converts to accommodate the labor and delivery with all the necessary equipment needed during that time.
- Women's Resource Center
- Administrative Offices
- Intensive Care Nursery
- Parents' Overnight Room
- Obstetrical Surgery Suite
- Staff Conference Room
- Male and Female Lockers
- Physician Lounge and Sleep Rooms
- Diagnostic Center
- Two Prelabor Testing Rooms and two Prelabor Exam Rooms.
- Staff Lounge
- Labor Lounge
- Quiet Room
- Four-Bay Labor Overflow Area
- Two Antepartum High Risk Rooms

FIRST FLOOR
- 34 Private Postpartum Rooms. Each has a vanity, a glider, an overstuffed chair that converts to a twin-size bed, an armoire, and French doors opening to a terrace lined with plants.
- Level I Nursery for Well Babies with 40 bassinets
- Nursing Offices
- Classroom and two Family Rooms

SAMPLE FACILITY FACT SHEET

GWINNETT WOMEN'S PAVILION

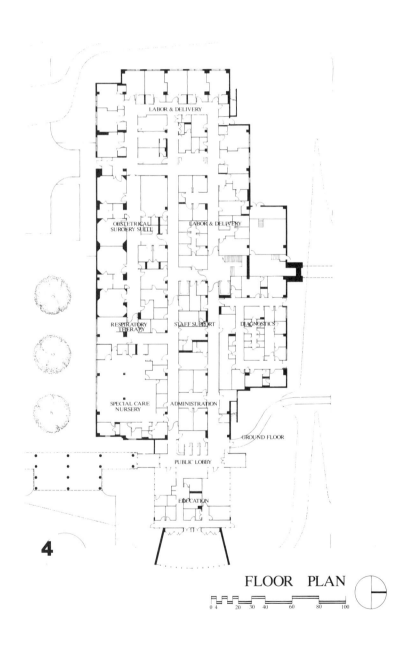

4

FLOOR PLAN

0 4 20 30 40 60 80 100

ARCHITECTURAL SPACE ISSUES

	Site	Public Spaces
Layout	Size: Adequacy, Expandability, Flexibility Placement of Building Circulation Accessibility: Patients, Staff, Visitors, Hospital Vehicles, Pedestrians, Handicapped Material Transportation Parking: Amount, Location	Location Space Circulation Accessibility Interdepartmental Relationships Privacy
Information / Wayfinding	Visibility of Arrival Point Signage: Size, Placement, Clarity, Contrast, Appearance, Consistency, Location, Display Staff Orientation Distinctiveness of Buildings Building Names and Addresses	Signage Communication Systems Information Technology Availability of Forms & Information Wayfinding Orientation
Technical	Security Strategy: Location, Visibility, Lighting, Alarm Zoning Restrictions Sound Control	Environmental Systems: Heating and Cooling, Humidity, Air Movement, Lighting, Ventilation, Air Quality Acoustics Security Strategy Control Access Smoke and Fire Protection
Furniture, Materials and Finishes	Plant Material and Hardscaping Landscaping Maintenance Durability	Location Ergonomics Accessibility Public Vending Durability Maintainability
Design Quality/ Amenities	Compatibility with Surroundings Amenities: Lunch and Recreation Areas Character of Environment Friendliness, Warmth, Welcoming, Reassuring Amenities: Plants, Seating	Maintenance Character of Environment Amenities Patient Friendliness

ARCHITECTURAL SPACE ISSUES

	Diagnostic & Treatment Areas	Patient Living Areas

Layout	Space
	Circulation
	Accessibility
	Relationship to Public
	    Areas/Spaces
	Transportation
	(ill/injured patients)
	Privacy
	  Space
	Circulation
		Location
		Space
		Circulation
		Accessibility
		Interdepartmental
		    Relationships
		Privacy

Information / Wayfinding	Signage Identifiability of Arrival Points Communication System/IT	Signage Identifiability Communication System/IT Wayfinding Orientation

Technical	Environmental Systems
	Security Strategy
	Repair, Condition
	Special Construction
	Isolation/Shielding from
	    Radiation, Utilities
	Material Transport: Supply,
	    Linen, Waste
	Smoke/Fire Protection
		Environmental
		  Systems
		Security Strategy
		Repair, Condition
		Material Transport: Supply,
		    Linen, Waste
		Smoke/Fire Protection

Furniture, Materials and Finishes	Durability Quality Cleanability Comfort Loading/Capacity Fire Protection	Durability Quality Cleanability Comfort Loading/Capacity Fire Protection

Design Quality /
Amenities
	Character of Environment
	Patient Friendliness
	Impact/Visibility of
	    Technological Equipment
	Territorial Control
	Color
	Scale of Environment
	Availability of Amenities
		Character of
		  Environment
		Patient Friendliness
		Impact/Visibility of
		    Equipment
		Territorial Control
		Color
		Scale of Environment
		Amenities

ARCHITECTURAL SPACE ISSUES

	Administrative and Office Areas	Support Areas
Layout	Size Location Circulation Storage Flexibility Privacy: Visual, Acoustical Interdepartmental Relationships Space	Location Locker Size/Location Comfort Storage Size Location Circulation Separation of Staff, Visitors, Patients and Materials Plan
Information / Wayfinding	Signage Communication System/IT Wayfinding	Signage Communication System/IT Wayfinding

Technical	Environmental
	   Systems
	Security Strategy
	Repair, Condition
	Material Transport: Supply,
	   Linen, Waste
	Smoke/Fire Protection
		Environmental
		   Systems
		Security Strategy
		Repair, Condition
		Material Transport: Supply,
		   Linen, Waste
		Smoke/Fire Protection

Furniture, Materials and Finishes	Location Ergonomics Accessibility Durability Cleanability Comfort Loading/Capacity Fire Protection	Location Accessibility Loading/Capacity Durability

Design Quality / Amenities	Character of
	   Environment
		Characteristics of Wall, Floor,
		   And Ceiling: Static-Free,
		   Washable, Nonslip, Color,
		   Wear, Cleaning
		   Characteristics

ISSUES WORKSHEET

Focus		Name	
Date		Firm	

TYPICAL ISSUES

QUESTIONS	RESOURCE	ISSUE TYPE	
	person or item	design	operational
		☐	☐
		☐	☐
		☐	☐
		☐	☐
		☐	☐
		☐	☐
		☐	☐
		☐	☐
		☐	☐
		☐	☐
		☐	☐
		☐	☐

HEALTHCARE FACILITY VISIT WORKSHEET

Name		Date	
Site		Keywords	
Area			

ISSUES CHECKLIST

OPERATIONAL/DESIGN ISSUES

CRITICAL ISSUES IN CONDUCTING FACILITY VISITS

SELECTING VISIT SITES

One of the most important steps in conducting healthcare facility visits is the selection of appropriate sites. However, there is no single source of information on healthcare facilities, and site selection is not an easy task. It is difficult to locate sites with comparable features in terms of workload, size, budget, operational facilities and physical features. Without this information, the tendency is to choose sites based on other criteria, such as location and proximity, or the presence of a friend or former coworker at specific host facilities.

However, depending on the nature of the facility visit, there are several resources that can be consulted for site selection. Some healthcare and design professional associations periodically publish guides and reference books which are helpful in selecting sites for facility visits. The following sources can be referred to before selecting specific facilities for field visits:

I.   NATIONAL HEALTHCARE ASSOCIATIONS

1.   American Hospital Association (AHA)
     AHA Resource Center, Chicago, (312) 280-6000

     AHA database for healthcare facilities in the state of Missouri.:
     Missouri Hospitals Profile. Listed price: $27.50.

     AHA Guide to locating healthcare facilities in the US.
     The listed facilities are classified according to the city/county with a coded format for the number of beds, admission fee, etc. Listed price: $195 for nonmembers and $75 for members.

     AHA Health Care Construction Database Survey.
     Contact Robert Zank at the AHA Division of Health Facilities Management, (312) 280-5910.

2.   Association of Health Facilities Survey Agency (AHFSA)
     Directory of the Association of Health Facilities Survey Agency.
     AHFSA, Springfield, IL.

3.   National Association of Health Data Organizations (NAHDO)
     Some states collect detailed hospital-level data. To obtain information on states with legislative mandates to gather hospital-level

data, contact Stacey Carman at 254 B N. Washington Street, Falls Church, VA 22046-4517, Telephone: (703) 532-3282, FAX: (703) 532-3593.

II. NATIONAL ASSOCIATIONS FOR DESIGN PROFESSIONALS

1. American Institute of Architects (AIA)
   AIA Academy on Architecture for Health
   1735 New York Avenue NW
   Washington, DC 20006
   (202) 626-7493 or (202) 626-7366, FAX (202) 626-7587
   To order AIA publications: (800) 365-2724

   Hospital Interior Architect.

   Hospital and Health Care Facilities, 1992.
   Listed price: $48.50 for nonmembers; 10% discount for members off listed price.

   Hospitals and Health Systems Review, July 1994.
   Listed price: $12.95 for nonmembers; 30 % discount for members off listed price.

   Hospital Planning.
   Listed price: $37.50 for nonmembers; 10% discount for members off listed price.

   Hospital Special Care Facility, 1993.

   Organizational Change: Transforming Today's Hospitals, January 1995.
   Listed price: $36.00 for nonmembers; 30% discount for members off listed price.

   Health Facilities Review (biannual), 1993.
   Listed price: $20 for nonmembers; $14 for members.

III. PERIODICALS DESCRIBING SPECIFIC HEALTHCARE FACILITIES

   Modern Healthcare.
   This national weekly business news magazine for healthcare management is published by Crain Communication, and holds annual

design awards. In conjunction with AIA Academy of Architecture for Health, this periodical announces annual competition and honors architectural projects that build on changes in healthcare delivery. Contact Joan Fitzgerald or Mary Chamberlain at 740 N. Rush Street, Chicago IL 60611-2590, (312) 649-5355.

American Hospital Association Exhibition of Architecture for Health, 1993.

For further information contact Robert Zank at the Division of Health Facilities Management, (312) 280-5910.

The Center for Health Design offers several resources.
They can be contacted at:
The Center for Health Design
4550 Alhambra Way
Martinez, CA 94553-4406
(510) 370-0345, Fax: (510) 228-4018.

Journal of Healthcare Design.
This journal illustrates 20-40 exemplary healthcare facilities in each annual issue.

Free list of previously-toured exemplary facilities (available by calling The Center).

Æsclepius.
Æsclepius is a newsletter discussing a range of design issues relevant to healthcare facilities.

TEAM BUILDING

Many people who conduct healthcare facility field visits use them as a way to build an ongoing design team. This is particularly true of designer-client-consultant teams who conduct visits early in a design project. According to organizational researcher and consultant J. Richard Hackman,[1] teams often spend too much time worrying about the "feel-good" aspects of interpersonal relationships and not enough time focusing on other key issues such as choosing the right people for the team, making roles and resources clear, specifying final products, and clarifying how the final product will be used.

Participants are often chosen because they are upper-level administrators or because they deserve the perk. It may not be clear what their function is on the visit or how they would contribute to any later decision making about the design project. Likewise, visit teams often don't know what resources are available to them: Can they visit national sites? Can they call on others to help prepare and distribute a visit report?

Some key team building steps include:

- Select visit participants with a clear idea of why they are participating and how they can contribute.

- Keep the team small; visit teams of more than seven or eight people are hard to manage.

- Provide each participant a clear role before, during and after the actual site visit, and negotiate this role to fit their interests and skills. Roles should be clearly differentiated and clear to all participants.

- Make the final product clear: simple photocopying and assembly of notes and photos taken during the visit; brief illustrated written report; videotape, etc.

- Clarify how the visit findings are to be used: what key decisions are the major focus?

---

[1] Hackman, J.R., "The design of work teams," Handbook of Organizational Behavior, ed. J.W Lorsch (Englewood Cliffs, NJ: Prentice-Hall, 1987): 315-343.

- Make resources clear.

- Give participants as much freedom from other tasks as possible during key times in planning, conducting and compiling the visit.

ROLES IN CONDUCTING FACILITY VISITS

There are several key roles in the process. Depending on the size of the team and the nature of the visit, each role may be taken on by a different person, or they may be combined.

LEADERSHIP TASKS:

- Restate current need and parameters of the design project.

- Develop some background information on the issues or setting types being investigated, and distribute to team members.

- Conduct a brainstorming meeting to understand the expertise, interests, values, and goals of each team member.

- Identify potential visit team members, and invite them.

- Summarize the goals of the design project, clarify how the field visit might advance these goals, and communicate these to the team.

- Identify roles for each team member.

- Develop a work plan and budget.

- Clarify the criteria for choosing sites.

- Prepare and/or review major documents: site-specific protocols; checklists and lists of questions and issues; information about each site being visited; overall plan for the visit; visit report; focus report.

- Conduct wrap-up meeting at each site.

- Conduct focus meeting on returning home.

SUPPORT TASKS:

- Assemble a few key articles or other documents to help the team understand the key issues in the setting types, processes or departments being visited.

- Identify potential sites, with some information about each site candidate so the leader and team can make final choices.
- Confirm with sites, and clarify what information the team will need in advance and what will be collected during the visit.

- Prepare draft materials (Background Brief, site information package, visit information, interview protocol) for review by the leader.

- Organize any trip logistics that are not done individually by participants: car rentals, hotel reservations, air tickets, etc.

- Write thank-you letters to site participants.

- Prepare a Draft Visit Report for review by the leader and team.

- Draft a Focus Report for review by the leader and the team.

FACILITATION TASKS:

When the team is attempting to get broad input into the process, such as when the team meets initially to set direction, it is often useful to have someone run the meeting who has the role of simply looking after the process of the meeting, rather than the content. He or she is charged with making sure that everyone is heard without prejudice, and that all positions are brought out. It often works poorly to have a senior manager in this role. Even if he or she has good facilitation skills, it is intimidating for many people to speak up in a meeting led by their boss.

Specific tasks:

- Conduct the initial brainstorming session that establishes the direction, issues and roles for the visit.

- Conduct any additional sessions where balanced participation is important to increasing the pool of ideas or getting "buy-in" from all team members.

RECORDER TASKS:

During the actual site visit, one or more people are typically charged with maintaining the "official" records of the visit (individuals may keep their own notes as well). This may include written notes, audio or video records, or photographs. If the team breaks up during the visit, a recorder should accompany each group.

Specific tasks include:

- Procure any required recording devices and supplies, such as cameras, tape recorders, paper forms, etc.

- Make records during the visit.

- Edit the record and assemble into a report.

TEAM PARTICIPANTS TASKS:

- Bring his or her goals and concerns to the attention of the team.

- If he or she is serving as a representative of a functional group or other constituency, such as the nursing staff, make sure that all interests of the group are represented.

- Immediately alert the team when communication problems occur, and particularly when jargon or technical issues prevent all participants from participating fully.

INTERVIEWING

Interviews vary greatly in the amount of control exercised by the interviewer in choosing the topic for discussion and in structuring the response. An intermediate level of control over topic and responses, often called a "structured interview," is usually appropriate in a facility visit. In a structured interview, the interviewer has an interview schedule which is a detailed list of questions or issues which serves as a general map of the discussion. However, the interviewer allows the respondent to answer in his or her own words and to follow his or her own order of questioning if desired. The interview is usually aided by walking through the setting or by having plans or other visual aids during seated sessions.

The use of fixed responses, in which respondents have to choose a "best" alternative among several presented, allows rapid analysis of results and may be appropriate if a large number of people are interviewed during a visit. The cost-effectiveness of interviews needs to be considered by the architect or manager when designing the process. Individual interviews are useful because people being questioned may be more forthcoming than if friends or colleagues are present. However, individual interviews are expensive. With scheduling, waiting time, running the interview, and coding, a brief individual interview may involve several hours or more of staff time.

In summary, interviews are valuable because people can directly communicate their feelings, motives and actions. However, interviews are limited by people's desire to be socially desirable or by their faulty memories, although these problems may not be too serious unless the questions are very sensitive.

CONCLUSIONS

Many healthcare organizations are looking to reduce their risk in designing and planning new facilities. There is no way to totally eliminate risk. The world is simply unpredictable, and will remain so. There are, however, ways to reduce risk: learning from the best and most innovative examples; looking at one's own operations in a critical way and considering new approaches that better fit changing conditions; seeing problems from new perspectives, and especially from those of customers such as patients and staff.

Unfortunately, many design processes do not do a good job at controlling risks, costs, and inefficiencies. A design project may have a big influence on the future of an organization, but critical operational and design decisions often receive too little attention. And problems or new ideas are often discovered very late in a design process, when they are difficult and costly to accommodate. It is not hard to understand the source of these difficulties. The crises of everyday life go on unabated during design and distract people from design, short-term politics continue, and many people are comfortable with what they already know. Many design team participants representing healthcare organizations want to reproduce their existing operation, even if they can recognize its flaws.

A healthcare design team is too often more like a raucous international meeting than like an effective task-oriented organization. Participants speak different professional languages, have different experiences, have different short-term objectives, hold different motivations for participating, and hold different values about what constitutes a successful project. The team may be far into a project before it understands the different viewpoints represented on the team.

A facility visit is a unique opportunity to address some of these problems. It provides an extended opportunity for a design or planning team to get together outside the pressures of daily life, to critically examine the operations of an excellent facility, to rethink its own ideas, and to build the basis of a team that may function for several years. It is often the longest uninterrupted time a team ever spends together, and the best chance to think in new ways.

A visit has three goals: to establish a situation for effective critical examination of state-of-the-art operations and facilities; to think about the project in new ways; and building a team. These goals are intertwined. A well-structured facility visit may help build a team more effectively than an artificial "feel-good" exercise of mountain climbing or simulated war games. A team that looks at a facility from different perspectives, and in which participants forcefully argue their viewpoint based on evidence from a common visit, can learn each other's strengths, preferences, and priorities quickly and in a way that builds a bond that is closely related to their own project.

Many teams, however, do not provide enough structure for either critical examination or team building. Critical examination requires an understanding of what key issues are to be examined and how they might apply to the current design problem. Team building requires that a team clearly establishes the role of each team member, makes the resources, process, and schedule clear, is explicit about the form and use of the final report, and establishes a common language.

Healthcare designers and consultants can develop better facility visits, but the responsibility for improving this practice rests with healthcare clients. For a visit to reach its potential, clients must demand an improved process, hold the organizer accountable-and be willing to pay for it. The healthcare client must see design and planning as a process open to mutual learning, and make it happen.

APPENDIX A:
BIBLIOGRAPHY

GENERAL POST-OCCUPANCY EVALUATION AND FACILITIES MANAGEMENT

Castor B (1990). Guide for Post-Occupancy Evaluations. Florida Department of Education.
This report identifies the sequence of events, time requirements, activities, and legal references necessary to successfully conduct a post-occupancy evaluation of individual school facilities for public education in Florida. A good source for program specialists who are assigned the responsibility of conducting a post-occupancy evaluation. Different kinds of questionnaires such as user, building, site, etc. are included.

Farbstein J, & Kantrowitz M (1985). Design Aesthetics and Postal Image-Building Visits. Real Estate and Building Department, United States Postal Service, Volume 1 (2-B).
This report is about visiting buildings to view the image of a broad sample of the existing US Postal Service building stock. At each post office, participants toured, photographed the building, interviewed, and rated the building on a specific scale. The building characteristics, rating scales, consultant comments on building image, and postmaster interview comments were entered into a data base for analysis. The reports of these analyses are included. More complete descriptions of the categories, along with illustrations, are also included.

Freidmann A, Zimring C, & Zube E (1978) Environmental Design Evaluation. New York: Plenum.
This book presents case studies and methods for evaluation of buildings and public spaces from several perspectives: setting, design process, social-historical context, proximate-environmental context.

Kernohan D, Gray J, Daish J, & Joiner D (1992). User Participation in Building Design and Management. Oxford: Butterworth-Heinemann Ltd.
This book discusses a generic participatory process for building evaluation, and provides a detailed "touring interview" methodology. It argues that the key to successful design is to integrate the knowledge of users and providers through shared experience, and that this can be accomplished during the building evaluation process.

Linttell C (1994) Health Care Facilities Condition Survey. Edmonton: Alberta (Canada) Public Works, Supply and Services Department, Health Facilities Project Division.
This survey form provides a comprehensive checklist for assessing the condition, suitability, and functionality of a healthcare facility. It focuses on several scales such as site, building and department. The package

includes forms, outline procedure manual and computer software for manipulating results and creating reports.

Preiser WFE, Rabinowitz H, & White W (1986) <u>Post-Occupancy Evaluation</u>. New York: Van Nostrand Reinhold.

<u>Post-Occupancy Evaluation</u> proposes a multi-level evaluation process depending on the team's goals and resources. Includes forms and methods that can be photocopied.

ADDITIONAL REFERENCES

Binder S (1992). <u>Strategic Corporate Facilities Management.</u> New York: McGraw-Hill.

COLLABORATIVE DESIGN

Leavitt J, & Sheine J (1990). "In-Between Architecture and Planning: Collaboration Instead of Opposition." In Miller W, O'Leary P, Oliver BP, & Urban S (Eds.), <u>The Architects of the In-Between: Proceedings of the 78th Meeting of Collegiate Schools of Architecture</u>. Washington, DC: ASCA Press.

This article presents the steps followed in designing a new "studio" at UCLA in 1989. The studio had several goals: to create a joint effort with the clients playing an active role in decision making, to familiarize students with different disciplines prior to the project, and most importantly, active involvement in policy making and design processes and informing and empowering the residents.

Sanoff H (1990). "Integrating Research and Design Participation: Applying Theory Z to Architecture." In Miller W, O'Leary P, Oliver BP, & Urban S (Eds.), <u>The Architects of the In-Between: Proceedings of the 78th Meeting of Collegiate Schools of Architecture</u>. Washington, DC: ASCA Press.

This article employs "Theory Z" which aims to establish an arena for collaboration between all parties involved in and influenced by design decisions. Case studies are utilized to illustrate the techniques characterizing this process.

Shibley R (1990). "Practitioner Reflections on Architectural Excellence." In Miller W, O'Leary P, Oliver B P, & Urban S (Eds.), <u>The Architects of the In-Between: Proceedings of the 78th Meeting of Collegiate Schools of Architecture</u>. Washington, DC: ASCA Press.

Shibley draws from the AIA's Design/Practice for the '90s program to analyze the major differences among the goals of architectural practice as they pertain to excellence. After reviewing the arguments of various professionals he concludes that all approaches are important in their own way and that the debate on excellence should be expanded to involve the stakeholders who occupy and use places.

Wagenknecht-Harte K (1989). <u>Site + Sculpture: The Collaborative Design Process</u>. New York: Van Nostrand Reinhold.
The main goal of this study is to emphasize the necessity and importance of collaboration in design, with a focus on urban design. The author forcefully argues that collaborative team designs have numerous advantages over single-discipline designs and provides both an historical overview and contemporary case studies to demonstrate the development of process guidelines.

ADDITIONAL REFERENCES

Schneekloth L, & Shibley R (1987). "Research/Practice: Thoughts on an Interactive Paradigm." In Shibley R (Ed.), <u>Proceedings of the American Association of Collegiate Schools of Architecture Annual Research Conference</u>. Washington, DC: AIA/ACSA Research Council.

Shibley R, & Schneekloth L (1988). "Risking Collaboration: Professional Dilemmas in Evaluation and Design." In <u>The Journal of Architectural and Planning Research</u> 5:4 (Winter).

BENCHMARKING

Adair C, & Murray C (1994). <u>Breakthrough Process Redesign</u>. New York: American Management Association.
This book is about business management issues, but talks about customer values, understanding minimum acceptable value, profiling customers' values, etc. Some sketches and figures are also provided. The authors talk about gathering data and how to conduct a customer value survey, and suggest a model of customer value. Later, there is some information about benchmarking, reasons, targets, and how to conduct "the benchmarking visit." Finally, there are some guidelines for written customer/client surveys/interviews and focus groups.

Boxwell R J (1994). <u>Benchmarking for Competitive Advantage</u>. New York: McGraw-Hill.
This book is written for people who want to learn what benchmarking is. The book contains lots of examples of how managers in a wide variety of industries have used benchmarking.

Gaskie M (1993). "Patients First." <u>Architecture</u> (March), 99-104.
Coverage of a mix of women's and PFC projects by Ratcliff, RTKL (Greater Baltimore Medical Center's OB/acute care addition), Bobrow/Thomas (St. Luke's Medical Center, Milwaukee), HDR (Lakeland Regional Medical Center), and NBBJ (Pomona Valley Hospital's women's center). With lots of plans and pictures for reference.

McNair C J (1992). <u>Benchmarking: A Tool for Continuous Improvement</u>.
New York: Harper Business.
This book is about different ways companies have used benchmarking to
gain competitive excellence and advantage.

Miller J, Meyer A, & Nakane J (1992). <u>Benchmarking Global Manufacturing.</u>
Homewood, IL: Business One Irwin.
This book is about providing benchmarking information and tools to
compare manufacturing strategies, operations and plans from various
industrial groups.

Patrick M, & Alba T (1994). "Health Care Benchmarking: A Team
Approach." <u>Quality Management in Health Care</u> 2 (2), 38-47.
In this paper, the authors argue that group benchmarking has significant
impact within the healthcare field as a means to measure quality, search
for better practices, and implement the necessary changes to meet
future healthcare challenges. The primary focus is on the utility of using
benchmarking and types of benchmarking. A benchmarking model for
hospitals is also suggested.

Watson G H (1992). <u>Strategic Benchmarking</u>. New York: Harper Business.
This book identifies better ways to use inter-business cooperation to
improve strategic planning and increase competitiveness. The first four
chapters describe the theory of benchmarking; the remaining chapters
apply benchmarking in a variety of situations. Major case studies of
benchmarking applications from Hewlett-Packard, Ford, General Motors,
and Xerox are included.

ADDITIONAL REFERENCES

Baum N (1992). "The Magical Medical Media Tour." <u>JAMA</u> 268 (16), 2168.

Clifford C (1992). "Professional Exchanges: Planning a Study Tour."
<u>Nursing-Times</u> 88 (15), 38-40.

Jardine G, & Lunda D (1993). "Predicting the Future: Master Planning for
Flexibility in School and College Utilities." <u>School and College</u>
(December), 11-16.

Golsby M (1992). "Four Steps to Success." <u>Security Management</u> (August),
53-54.

Goldberg AM, & Pegels CC (1984). <u>Quality Circles in Health Care
Facilities: A Model for Excellence</u>. Rockville, MD: Aspen Systems Corp.

Monroe L (1992). "What Do Facility Managers Need?" <u>Buildings</u> 86 (October), 38.

Shactman D (1993). "Smart Financial Management of Medical Office Space." <u>Healthcare Financial Management </u>(June 5), 81-85.

Spendolini M (1992). <u>The Benchmarking Book</u>. New York: American Management Association.

Sraeel I (1991). "Defining the Facilities Manager of the `90s." <u>Buildings</u> 85 (July), 40-45.

Umeno S (1992). "Facility Management: Making the Best Use of Facilities." <u>Japan 21st </u>(October 3), 63.

DESIGN GUIDES AND THE DESIGN PROCESS

Beaven L, & Dry D (1983). <u>Architect's Job Book</u>. London: RIBA Publications.
The <u>Job Book</u> establishes the procedures to be followed for a model pattern of working and provides a checklist of key management activities. It aids the building industry and the associated professions in coping with the management of design and building processes.

Borzo G (1992). "Market Memo: patient-focused hospitals begin reporting good results." <u>Health Care Strategic Management</u> (August), 17-22.
A good overall look at patient-focused care restructuring with Mercy Hospital, San Diego, as the prime example.

Carpman J, & Grant M (1993). <u>Design That Cares: Planning Health Facilities for Patients and Visitors</u> (Second ed.). Chicago: American Hospital Association Publishing.
This book is written for designers, administrators, architects, engineers, interior designers, healthcare delivery staff, etc. who deal with healthcare and healthcare design. The book has three parts: background information on current societal and demographic trends and their impact on healthcare; specific information on how facility design can aid patients and visitors; user participation in the design process as a way for design decision makers to build on general principles by gathering information specific to the issues at hand.

Cohen U (1993) <u>Contemporary Environments for People with Dementia</u>. Baltimore: Johns Hopkins.
Provides an overview of principles for design and research into facilities for people with Alzheimer's disease and other dementias. Provides many examples.

Cohen U, & Weisman G (1991) <u>Holding on to Home</u>. Baltimore: Johns Hopkins.
Provides a user-oriented approach to the design of facilities for patients with Alzheimer's disease, with several case studies.

<u>Facilities Planning News</u> (1993). "Sentara Norfolk General Hospital's River Pavilion." In <u>Facilities Planning News</u> (July).
Description of the Sentara project and summary of the Booz-Allen Model.

Flexner WA, Berkowitz EN, & Brown M (1981). <u>Strategic Planning in Health Care Management</u>. Rockville, MD: Aspen Systems Corp.
This book combines previously published healthcare articles that address strategic planning and its management disciplines.

Gregerson J (1993). "The Ideal Patient Treatment." <u>Building Design & Construction</u> (November), 36-39.
Johns Hopkins Hospital stitches together a medical experience with its new 420,000-sq.-ft. Outpatient Center.

Jenna K (1986). "Toward the Patient-Driven Hospital. " <u>Healthcare Forum</u> (May/June), 9-14, 17-18.
A good presentation of the patient-focused Planetree model at CPMC.

Klein B, & Platt A (1989). <u>Health Care Facility Planning & Construction</u>. New York: Van Nostrand Reinhold.
This book is about providing assistance for all types of healthcare facility construction projects and for all types of persons involved in planning such projects or studying the process of building such facilities. Chapter eight covers the topic of "Evaluation of Existing and New Facilities and Operations." The issues stressed in this chapter are: "Who should do the evaluation?"; "When should the evaluation be done?"; "What should be evaluated?"; "What is to be built?"; and a checklist for "How to survey an existing facility."

Lamarche D (1993). "Preoperative Structured Patient Education." <u>Canadian-Nurse</u> 89 (4), 38-41.
This article describes the factors that motivated the nursing staff of the cardiac unit at the Royal Victoria Hospital in Montreal to revise the length of the pre-operative waiting period; the level of pre-operative anxiety with current patient teaching practices; and the lack of available resources. The reorganization of the teaching program was based upon the previously described factors combined with a review of the literature that demonstrated the impact of pre-operative anxiety, emotional support and psycho-educational interventions upon the client's recovery.

Malkin, J (1992) <u>Hospital Interior Architecture</u>. New York: Van Nostrand Reinhold.

This book explores research on the relationship between the environment and healing, surveys a wide range of outstanding facilities, and provides design guidelines on creating healing environments for specific patient populations: children, elderly, critical care, cancer, chemical dependency, rehabilitation, neonates, perinatal, and others. It also includes chapters on wayfinding design, psychology of color, adulatory care settings, psychiatric risk management tactics, and congregate care housing. Includes numerous illustrations and color plates.

Olds AR, & Daniel PD (1987). <u>Child Health Care Facilities</u>. Washington, DC: Association for the Care of Children's Health.

A good source for all those who may be involved in the design of new construction and/or renovation of an entire healthcare facility where infants and children receive care: administrators, hospital trustees, architects, designers, planners, building contractors, parents, nurses, physicians, child life specialists, etc. The book has two parts: "Design Guidelines" and "Literature Outline." In the "Design Guidelines" section, children's healthcare facilities are investigated as general, external and medical spaces. Literature review is done for the same categories.

Valins MS (1993). <u>Primary Health Care Centers</u>. New York: John Wiley & Sons, Inc.

This book is a consolidation of ideas and guidelines about critical design issues in primary healthcare facilities.

ADDITIONAL REFERENCES

Belsey RE (1986). <u>The Physician's Office Laboratory</u>. Oradell, NJ: Medical Economics Books.

Bosker G (1987). "Architecture as an Asset in Health Care." <u>Architecture</u> (January), 48-53.

Brauer R (1986). <u>Facilities Planning: The User Requirements Method</u>. New York: American Management Association.

Cox A, & Groves P (1981). <u>Design for Health Care</u>. Fakenham, Norfolk: Butterworths.

Cushman RF, & Perry S (1983). <u>Planning, Financing, and Constructing Health Care Facilities</u>. Rockville, MD: Aspen Systems Corp.

Konz S (1985). <u>Facility Design</u>. New York: John Wiley & Sons.

Lewis D (1991). "Turning Rust into Gold: Planned Facility Management." Public Administration Review (November-December), 494-502.

Malkin J (1982). The Design of Medical and Dental Facilities. New York: Van Nostrand Reinhold.

Malkin J (1990). Medical and Dental Space Planning for the 1990s. New York: Van Nostrand Reinhold.

Pegels C, & Rogers KA (1988). Strategic Management of Hospitals and Health Care Facilities. Rockville, MD: Aspen Publishers.

Porter D (1982). Hospital Architecture: Guidelines for Design and Renovation. Ann Arbor, MI: Aupha Press.

Rostenberg B (1987). Design and Planning for Freestanding Ambulatory Care Facilities. Chicago: American Hospital Association.

Schwartz M (1989). Designing and Building Your Professional Office. Oradell, NJ: Medical Economics Books.

Smith J (1993). "Patient Oriented Care: New Focus for the 90's. " Article (23), 2-5.

World Health Organization (1983). Approaches to Planning and Design of Health Care Facilities in Developing Areas. Geneva: WHO Offset Publications.

APPENDIX B:
EXEMPLARY MICRO-CASES

Several visits were conducted during the preparation of this guide to help develop and test the visit methodology. Two of these are presented below.

DESIGNING A NEW HOSPITAL FOR THE UNITED KINGDOM

Tour of California Hospitals by a Healthcare Trust of United Kingdom National Health Service, Bruce Nepp, Anshen + Allen Architects

In this case a design team was concerned with creating a new hospital in the UK, and visited some state-of-the-art US facilities to learn about the design and operational implications of patient-focused care.

PREPARATION

■ TASK 1. SUMMARIZE THE DESIGN PROJECT
The proposed new hospital is located in Northern England. Due to recent changes in government policy, the new facility will allow the client to utilize design options of the client's choice rather than forcing them to employ the standardized hospital design prepared by the government some 20 years ago.

The client hopes to construct a new hospital in the UK that incorporates best of British and American operational and design concepts. The design professionals will be the Anglo-American firm of Anshen & Dyer Associates. The construction will be divided into two phases. The first phase will cost nearly $300 million. The first phase replaces the existing inpatient hospital.

■ TASK 2. PREPARE BACKGROUND BRIEF
Whereas the majority of the phase one project involves replacement of the inpatient services, the building must consider and support a trend toward decreasing inpatient services and increasing outpatient services. Such areas of consideration will include:

• High technology medical services and information technology.

• Outpatient facilities.

■ TASK 3. PREPARE DRAFT WORK PLAN AND BUDGET
The administrative staff of the hospital prepared a budget for the tour. However, the budget did not include sufficient reimbursements for all of the preparation tasks. The client asked that the architect make all logis-

tical arrangements, with the exception of air travel. The architect was given approximately two weeks to make these arrangements.

■ TASK 4. CHOOSE AND INVITE PARTICIPANTS
The client formed policy task forces for each unit involved in the design of the project (e.g., Surgical Institute, Family Institute, Clinical Support, etc.). A member from each task force was selected to participate in the tour. The client intentionally did not select the chairpersons of the task forces. The touring participants included consultants (specialist physicians), nurses, and clinical support representatives. Also included was the facility's project manager.

■ TASK 5. CONDUCT TEAM ISSUES SESSION
The client did not conduct a team issues session, which would have required each task force to develop its own list of issues for review. These lists were not formally consolidated into the Issues Worksheet format as presented in this report. The final format of the Issues Worksheets was unavailable at the time of this tour. However, the field data have been transcribed into the suggested format.

■ TASK 6. IDENTIFY POTENTIAL SITES AND START FACILITY VISIT PACKAGE
California was selected as the tour site due to the proximity of Anshen Dyer Associates offices (Anshen + Allen) at San Francisco and Los Angeles. Also, California has been the birthplace of many major healthcare trends. Several sites were selected based on the facilities' use of patient-focused care concepts, areas of expertise, and/or because they were recently constructed. The selected team visited nine facilities. One facility consisted of an all-day seminar on patient-focused care concepts at a host hospital.

■ TASK 7. SCHEDULE SITES AND CONFIRM AGENDA
The architect made all the arrangements for local transportation and accommodations and scheduled visits with the host facilities.

■ TASK 8. PREPARE FIELD VISIT PACKAGE
a) Visitor information package: The architect prepared this document in addition to the tour logistics.

b) Visit itineraries: The tour participants arrived from Britain on the day before the facilities visits. The architect arranged a sightseeing tour of San Francisco and gave them maps and tourist brochures. (This was very effective at breaking the ice and creating an initial sense of camaraderie.)

c) Site information package: The architect prepared the site information package based on the information provided by the host facilities. In the case where the architect designed the project, the firm's own materials were used. Since each participant developed his/her own issues list, the current form of the Issues Worksheets was not used. The tour sites were chosen for specific concepts or areas of expertise; few, if any, excel in all disciplines that were represented by the tour group. Last-minute appointments were scheduled to provide peer-to-peer interviews.

FACILITY FIELD VISIT

■ TASK 9. CONDUCT FIELD VISIT
The tour group traveled together via bus. An architect accompanied them throughout the trip to make introductions and provide logistical support. In most of the cases, the architect was able to provide an initial orientation to the facility. In several cases, a healthcare representative of the facility provided the orientation. As an example, a Site Visit Worksheet has been produced for the Mt. Diablo Medical Center (MDMC) tour. MDMC recently completed its new wing, which includes a birthing center, patient care units, and education center. In addition, the group toured MDMC's freestanding day surgery center. The tour group was given a general overview by Anshen + Allen, the project's architect, then the group was subdivided and sent to their areas of expertise. In each case, a subgroup met with the manager of the department. In some cases, physicians were also made available.

FINDINGS

■ TASK 10. ASSEMBLE DRAFT VISIT REPORT
The notes of each participant were assembled to focus on which aspects of the US experience could be imported to their hospital, and which should be avoided. Debriefing sessions were held each night to identify conclusions and issues. The architect attended these debriefings to help "interpret" US practices, systems, and technology. In addition, it was helpful for the architect to learn more about its client and their goals and objectives.

■ TASK 11. CONDUCT FOCUS MEETING
The visit team chose to share its visit with collegeageus via slide several presentations. Detailed presentations were made to the task forces comprising tour participants; a more general presentation was made by the entire group to the hospital at-large on two afternoons.

■ TASK 12. PREPARE FOCUS REPORT
The slide show and verbal focus reports were prepared by each visit participant, who was responsible for representing and reporting back to a department or functional group. This was effective in maintaining a high level of attention by each participant.

■ TASK 13. USE DATA TO INFORM DESIGN
The tour group members are representatives of the Task Forces who were programming and designing the departments or functional groups, and actively use their experience to inform design.

HEALTHCARE FACILITY VISIT WORKSHEET

Name	Day Surgery	Date	
Site	Mt Diablo Medical Center	Keywords	Surgery, day surgery, operating theatres
Area			

ISSUES CHECKLIST

1. Types and quantities of procedures performed and number and scheduling of operating theaters

2. Staffing ratios

3. Job descriptions

4. Pre-admissions procedures

5. Recovery hours/After hours

6. Review public spaces

7. Review medical equipment

8. Use of information technology and off-site interface

1. Procedures and quantities on a separate handout from host

2. Three theatres: they don't schedule by sessions but by blocks of time

3. Job descriptions supplied to tour by host

4. Primarily physician work-up with phone contact

5. 7:00 am-5:30 pm--"after hours" scheduled. Only rarely not anticipated.

6. Pleasant, quiet

OPERATIONAL/DESIGN ISSUES

FOCUSING ON INTERIORS

North Tower Interior Design Project, Lynn Befu, Anshen + Allen Architects and Interiors

In these facility visits the client was interested in learning about the durability and appearance of a specific interior finish, and in understanding alternative layouts and furnishings of cafeterias and gift shops.

PREPARATION

■ TASK 1. SUMMARIZE THE DESIGN PROJECT
Project description: County Medical Center. A 300,000-square-foot replacement facility, including a new main entrance and lobby, three floors of nursing units (ICUs, Med/Surg, Neurosurgical, Pediatrics, NICU and LDRs), Diagnostic Imaging, 12-room Surgical Suite, and two-room Cath Lab. Also includes Admitting, Gift Shop, Coffee Shop, and a four-floor circulation link. The client has also asked the designers to handle the arrangements for conducting facility visits.

Scope of services: Full architectural and interior design, including limited interior architecture, selection of materials and finishes, selection of furnishings, window coverings, and cubicle curtains.

Interior design goals: The client's goals were to create an attractive, but highly functional facility. The team saw the interior design as an opportunity to recognize the civic importance of the hospital, which has the ability to reach a large and diverse population. The following are some major interior design goals for the project:

*   To develop a building which is easy to use by employing colors, artwork, and signage to enhance and clarify the overall building organization and circulation and by acknowledging and addressing the varying physical requirements of a broad population base.

*   To create a light and refreshing interior design which is connected to the landscaped greenery of the plaza, terraces, balconies and other outdoor spaces by framing and directing views, and by careful development of lighting and other interior materials and colors.

*   To create memorable and enduring spaces which are calm, comfortable, and professional and which look better for longer.

- To support the community through both education and the promotion of wellness and the celebration of the arts.

- To support the operations of the staff by the attentive development of interior systems and schemes which streamline function and maintenance requirements and which attempt to improve occupational safety for all.

■ TASK 2. PREPARE BACKGROUND BRIEF
Critical materials: Due to the goals for low maintenance and high durability, the designers proposed the use of terrazo linoleum flooring. Background information on local installations, life cycle costs, and maintenance were distributed.

Public spaces: Several public spaces were identified and named as priorities for site visits.

■ TASK 3. PREPARE DRAFT WORK PLAN AND BUDGET
Target length of the visit: One eight-hour day was identified as appropriate.

Arrangements: The designers elected to identify possible sites, contact hosts, and pre-tour.

■ TASK 4. CHOOSE AND INVITE PARTICIPANTS
Facility visit participation included eight active team members:

- Medical Center Director, Professional and Support Services
- County Assistant Program Manager
- County Design Coordinator
- Interior Designers (3)

■ TASK 5. CONDUCT TEAM ISSUES SESSION
Because the layman's approach to interior design can be somewhat subjective, two exercises were employed to develop a "common language" which both designers and clients understood and which would serve as an introduction to the methodology of viewing visit sites.

Client values exercise: An exercise in which team members individually identify the desired qualities for the hospital, including global and departmental areas and specific rooms. Key questions included: 1) How should someone feel in a space? 2) What should they remember about a space?

Color exercise: An interactive exercise designed to discuss the effects of color distribution, relationship, scale, values and tone. This was meant to be a fun and educational foray into one of the more familiar aspects of interior design, while providing a more sophisticated approach to the use of color.

■ TASK 6. IDENTIFY POTENTIAL SITES AND START FACILITY VISIT PACKAGE
Targeted sites included public areas and hospital corridors, as well as installations of the critical materials. The designers brainstormed sites including hospitals, corporate campuses, retail areas, and outdoor plazas and terraces. Local installations of linoleum and high technology wall covering were provided by manufacturers' representatives.

Potential sites were limited to within the Bay Area; however, due to the allowable eight-hour window, the San Jose-San Francisco corridor became the area of concentration. Over 30 sites were identified and pre-toured during working and weekend hours. The final choice included: a) Peninsula Shopping Center; b) Cafe; c) Computer Campus Inc.; d) University Hospital. Contacts were initiated and preliminary visit times set up with these four facilities.

Sites were short-listed based on a combination of relative location and ability to address the goals of the visit. Careful attention was paid to logistics: 1) to cover the optimum distance while keeping driving time to a minimum; 2) to provide adequate observation time while shepherding a group of eight people; and 3) as our coffee shop was key public space, an effort was made to lunch in an appropriate and enjoyable spot.

■ TASK 7. SCHEDULE SITES AND CONFIRM AGENDA
The itinerary was roughed out. Desired arrival times and durations were confirmed with contacts and minor adjustments due to host requirements were made. In order to "corral" comments for the group's benefit, it was decided that the team should travel together. The county provided access to a van.

■ TASK 8. PREPARE FIELD VISIT PACKAGE
a) Visitor information package: see attached package.

b) Visit itineraries: See attached Site Visits Itinerary Sheet.

c) Site information package: In hindsight, the inclusion of a key photograph, site plan, and basic project information would have been beneficial. However, since each site was pre-toured, the checklists have been transcribed for each site.

FACILITY FIELD VISIT

TASK 9. CONDUCT FIELD VISIT
Orientation: During the first leg of travel, the purpose of the field visits was reiterated and the intended agenda for the first stop was outlined.

Interviews: Because one of the purposes relied on gathering subjective impressions of the interior, the team was asked first to form their own impressions. Then informal interviews were provided in most of the spaces.

Documentation: In addition to the field visit packages, the three designers became the designated recorders; one kept notes, one was responsible for photographs, and one color-matched key materials and paint colors.

Management: In order to alleviate the logistics of shepherding the group, one designer acted as the group leader (keeping sight of the purpose and process), while another acted as tour guide (facilitating travel and con- tacts).

FINDINGS

■ TASK 10. ASSEMBLE DRAFT VISIT REPORT
All field visit packages were collected for the record. We displayed photographs of the sites visited on boards for quick reference. Site- specific material and color samples were gathered and labeled for reference. Notes were used as follow-up questions at the focus meeting.

■ TASK 11. CONDUCT FOCUS MEETING
Round robin: An immediate follow-up meeting was conducted the day after the field visits. General impressions and lessons learned were recorded and compiled in a short Focus Report.

■ TASK 12. PREPARE FOCUS REPORT
The following key issues resulted from the facility visits:

•   Simplicity: Keep it simple, not complex or trendy.

- Choice: Need to provide a variety of areas where people can gather, have a sense of privacy and feel safe and secure, without compromising security. Variety can improve procession through spaces.

- Architectural development: Good interior spaces require integration of finishes with "architectural" detail. Curves soften boxy spaces. Contrast provides interest.

■ TASK 13. USE DATA TO INFORM DESIGN
The following critical observations will feed the design project:

- Warmth of materials: The use of familiar materials such as wood and carpet go a long way in humanizing a space; judicious use of harder materials (such as stainless steel and granite) need not be avoided, and when combined with "warm" materials (such as wood, carpet and art) can result in an interesting and inviting space.

- Color palette: Preferred palettes had warm neutral backgrounds, with soft accent colors.

- Lighting and acoustics: Natural light tends to lighten and soften the impact of color. In addition to acoustical ceilings, carpet contributes substantially to the "quietness" of a space.

HEALTHCARE FACILITY VISIT WORKSHEET

Name	Lynn Befu	Date	
Site	Computer Campus	Keywords	
Area	Lobbies		

ISSUES CHECKLIST

How does the LOBBY meet our common values?
1. Calming/comforting
2. Quiet
3. Classy/classic, grand and important
4. Comfortable
5. User-friendly
6. Informative
7. Welcoming
8. Reassuring, professional
8. Civic

How does this space meet our global values?
1. Easy to use
2. Light and airy
3. Lasting/Enduring
4. Calm
5. Artwork (and impacts on surrounding environment)
6. Safe
7. Lifegiving/Uplifting/Therapeutic
8. Inside out (awareness of outside)
9. High-touch

Are the acoustics appropriate?
Note any additional materials?
How large is the signage?
Is the space warm or cool?

OBSERVATIONS
Acoutics not good: loud echoes

Bld 3--NO!
Bld 6--Too neutral, needs artwork
Bld 1--strong colors

somewhat confusing interior spaces

Not enough artwork anywhere.

Too corporate for us!

Liked the paint/ tile combination in Building 6

Food service in Bld 4 was most efficient: Who did the installation?

OPERATIONAL/DESIGN ISSUES

Is too much maintenance required for our hospital?

Does reception double as a security control point?

We recommend wearing comfortable walking shoes!

Meet	7:45 am	Annex Building Parking Lot County Medical Center
Travel	7:45 - 8:15 am	
Site Visit	8:15 - 10:00 am	Computer Campus, Inc. Silicon Valley
Meet with	Project Manager 1 Project Manager 2 To view: Lobby spaces	 Cafeteria Material: Xorel
Travel	10:00 - 10:45 am	
Site Visit	10:45 - 12:00 am	University Hospital Peninsula
	To view:	Public Corridors & Gift Shop Children's Hospital
Meet with:	Director of Interior To view:	Design Anshen + Allen Public Corridors Typical Waiting Room Gift Shop
Travel	12:00- 12:15 am	
Lunch	12:15 - 1:15 pm	Cafe
Site Visit	1:15 - 2:00 pm	Peninsula Shopping Center
Travel	2:00 - 2:25 pm	
Site visit	2:25 - 2:45 pm	Computer Facility Foster City
	To view:	Cafeteria flooring Material: Marmoleum
Site visit	2:45 - 3:25 pm	Corporate Headquarters Meet with: Director Facilities
	To view:	Lobby & Cafeteria Material: Xorel
Travel	3:25 - 4:00 pm	4:00 pm estimated arrival at County Medical Center